The Hour of Birth

To explore the impact of psychoanalytic ideas and contemporary visual artists upon each other, this volume examines the aesthetics of the sublime as an allegory for psychic birth.

Through the lens of a radically intersubjective psychoanalytic theory, Civitarese reinvents the Freudian notion of sublimation. He theorizes that the aesthetic of the sublime reflects the internal process of establishing a space of thought through the gradual differentiation of subject and object. Supported by numerous artworks by contemporary artists – from Serra to Kapoor, and Wei to Kiefer – the volume attends to questions such as: How does the psyche come into being? Why can beauty be considered necessary for life? How does what we experience as "simply" beautiful differ from the aesthetic experience of what is called "sublime"? In this way, Civitarese forges a conceptual tool that enables readers to weave together psychoanalytic theory and aesthetics.

Drawing on a deep understanding of both the latest psychoanalytic thinking and artistic practices, this book will appeal to all psychoanalysts and psychotherapists interested in art and questions of psychic development.

Giuseppe Civitarese, MD, PhD, is a psychiatrist and training and supervising analyst of the Italian Psychoanalytic Society (SPI), and a member of the American Psychoanalytic Association (APsaA) and of the International Psychoanalytic Association (IPA). He lives and is in private practice, in Pavia, Italy.

THE NEW LIBRARY OF PSYCHOANALYSIS
General Editor: Anne Patterson

The *New Library of Psychoanalysis* is published by Routledge Mental Health in association with the *Institute of Psychoanalysis*, London.

The purpose of the book series is:

- to advance and disseminate ideas in psychoanalysis amongst those working in psychoanalysis, psychotherapy and related fields
- to facilitate a greater and more widespread appreciation of psychoanalysis in the general book-reading public
- to provide a forum for increasing mutual understanding between psychoanalysts and those in other disciplines
- to facilitate communication between different traditions and cultures within psychoanalysis, making some of the work of continental and other non-English speaking analysts more readily available to English-speaking readers, and increasing the interchange of ideas between British and American analysts.

The *New Library of Psychoanalysis* published its first book in 1987 under the editorship of David Tuckett, who was followed by Elizabeth Bott Spillius, Susan Budd, Dana Birksted-Breen and Alessandra Lemma. The Editors, including the current Editor, Anne Patterson, have been assisted by a considerable number of Associate Editors and readers from a range of countries and psychoanalytic traditions. The present Associate Editors are Susanne Calice, Katalin Lanczi and Anna Streeruwitz.

Under the guidance of Foreign Rights Editors, a considerable number of the *New Library* books have been published abroad, particularly in Brazil, Germany, France, Italy, Peru, Spain and Japan. The *New Library of Psychoanalysis* has also translated and published several books by continental psychoanalysts and plans to continue the policy of publishing books that express as clearly as possible a variety of psychoanalytic points of view. The *New Library of Psychoanalysis* has published books representing all three schools of thought in British psychoanalysis, including a particularly important work edited by Pearl King and Riccardo Steiner, '*The Freud-Klein Controversies*

1941-45', expounding the intellectual and organisational controversies that developed in the British psychoanalytical Society between Kleinian, Viennese and 'middle group' analysts during the Second World War.

The *New Library of Psychoanalysis* aims for excellence in psychoanalytic publishing. Submitted manuscripts are rigorously peer-reviewed in order to ensure high standards of scholarship, clinical communications, and writing.

For a full list of all the titles in the New Library of Psychoanalysis main series as well as both the New Library of Psychoanalysis 'Teaching Series' and 'Beyond the Couch' subseries, please visit the Routledge website.

The Hour of Birth

Psychoanalysis of the Sublime and Contemporary Art

Giuseppe Civitarese

Routledge
Taylor & Francis Group
LONDON AND NEW YORK

Designed cover image: THE HOUR OF BIRTH, 1901/02, Alfred Kubin (Leitmeritz/Litoměřice 1877–1959 Zwickledt), Pen and India ink wash, spray technique on cadastral paper, 25.5 × 30.6 cm.

First published in English 2026
by Routledge
4 Park Square, Milton Park, Abingdon, Oxon OX14 4RN

and by Routledge
605 Third Avenue, New York, NY 10158

Routledge is an imprint of the Taylor & Francis Group, an informa business

Translated by Giuseppe Civitarese, revised by Ian Harvey

British Library Cataloguing-in-Publication Data
A catalogue record for this book is available from the British Library

ISBN: 978-1-032-76530-3 (hbk)
ISBN: 978-1-032-76528-0 (pbk)
ISBN: 978-1-003-47890-4 (ebk)

DOI: 10.4324/9781003478904

Typeset in Bembo
by KnowledgeWorks Global Ltd.

Contents

List of Illustrations

Acknowledgements

I would like to thank Giuseppe Varchetta for kindly allowing me to reproduce some of his photos of works by Anish Kapoor.

Foreword

Art Is Either Sublime, or It Is Not Art

Here we have a psychoanalyst who not only has a good ear but also a good eye. He listens but he also looks. What is more, he has faith – faith in the art of the paintings he contemplates and faith in the verbal art he himself practises – psychoanalysis. In this book – which is a tribute to the way in which contemporary art is in harmony with the classically inspired rhetoric of the sublime, and with the Freudian-inspired concept of sublimation – Giuseppe Civitarese daringly interweaves two passions, or, one might even say, two faiths. Or put more simply perhaps, he combines two "love's bodies", two faces of the matter that sustains him, the food of which he partakes with such passion and rigour, namely, psychoanalysis and art.

The theme is "birth", as the title announces. Or rather, the "hour of birth" – birth as the introduction to the idea of time, and as the perspective of generation which in itself sets up the arc between before and after. In truth, to those who make themselves aware of it (which not everyone can do or wants to do), the here and now, the focal point, and the timely dart of birth are daily recurring themes in the experience of living. As we learn from John Keats, "That which is *creative* must create itself". These are the words of a poet Giuseppe Civitarese knows very well, and one he duly quotes in this book in recognition of his capacity to provide enlightenment.

It would be wonderful if we could say, modifying only slightly the young poet's deliberately apodictic assertion: If you are alive, you create yourself every day. By which I mean, it would be great if the experience of living were there for each of us in the thrill of a birth that happens day after day, in the daily act of self-creation. But, as we learn from Virginia Woolf, life, quotidian existence is made up not only of "moments of being" but also of an opaque fabric which, if anything, impairs the workings of our machine of perception. And it is precisely because the miracle of being born does not happen every day – certainly at least not to everyone – that we need doctors to take care of a psyche that is not always able to take flight, a soul not always capable of finding itself, of knowing itself.

Running alongside the theme of birth is that of artistic creation; that is, of another experience of birth – when the artist gives birth to the work, which always takes place beyond him, outside his reach, and which leaves him stranded on the shores of dejection. Because if there is such a thing as felicity of expression, if it does exist, and the artist undoubtedly is acquainted with it, that same artist is also familiar with the black hole of anguish. And perhaps it is precisely in this hole, more than anywhere else, that s/he finds *jouissance.*

Of course, the "work" that is born does not come into the world in the same way as the "creature" does. The artist is not the "mother" of the work in exactly the same way as the mother is the mother of a creature. Artists know this. And if they, in their own way, know the maternal side of creation, and experience its pangs, they also bear the burden of alienation and dispossession that the work forces upon them as it comes into being. Clearly, it is true that in our lexicon the verbs "to be born", "to generate", "to make", "to produce", and the nouns "work" and "product" collide with and brush up against each other in the shared field of the language we speak. The fact is certainly interesting in itself; by which I mean that the discourse of art and on art ends up, even against one's will, blending with that of generation and birth, going so far as to share ambiguous borders with it; to the point where it is impossible to really distinguish clearly between the two. Indeed, the two find themselves treading contiguous territories in acrimonious tension with each other, leading to a certain unease. It is also for this reason that centuries ago now – to be precise, at the beginning of the 19th century, a century as bourgeois, economically driven, and violent as any – there were artists who urgently advocated the need to find another idea of beauty; and they resorted to a winding line as the key to understanding modern beauty. Poets, painters, philosophers – the best, the greatest – believed in all conscience that beauty could, indeed should, verge on the hideous.

They believed that one could no longer think of the beautiful and the good as being in agreement, as dictated by the ancient principle of *Kalokagathìa*. And then there was a woman by the name of Mary Shelley who indeed created, gave birth to, generated Frankenstein. And, as you will remember, the confusion between the monster and the person who created him is already built into the name. It is as if the creature and the creator were one.

Here, too, poetry helps us. And once again it is the poet John Keats who comes to our aid, by reminding us in his *Ode on a Grecian Urn* that "truth is beauty, beauty truth". I have purposely reversed the order, because ultimately it doesn't matter. By which I mean that the sequence can be altered; the point is not whether truth or beauty comes first. The important thing to understand is that beauty must come to capture truth; and the truth is that ugliness, anguish, death, pain, and separation exist. All this is not simply *reality*; it is the *truth*. No more platonic illusions of celestial harmonies or any old artificial paradise. Art in an age of poverty cannot avert its eyes from poverty. Not that the artist should "illustrate' it, or "decorate" it, or even less console us by spouting mournful end-of-the-world rhetoric. This is not what art does. This is not what we ask of the artist. Nor is this what Giuseppe Civitarese asks of the artist.

True, as a psychoanalyst Civitarese is interested in art – after all, hasn't that always been the case with psychoanalysts? Surely from the very beginning, those who were interested in the human psyche were fascinated by art. By painting, by poetry. By myth, in all its varied forms? So Civitarese inherits that tradition, and he does so seriously, out of a deep sense of responsibility towards his science, his doctrine, and the heritage of knowledge that he continues to enrich in this way, namely, by lending an ear to that very special energy of life and thought that courses through the work of art. In this sense, for him, works of art are at their core "political". He confirms this in this book.

In what sense and how, you may ask? For one thing, in the sense that, as always in great human creative works, what can be admired is not only the concrete application of a talent, which in itself explains nothing; how can we explain why Turner paints the way he does? Nor is it about execution at the highest level of *expertise* perfectly suited to the purpose. Art is not only this: it is more, indeed there is an added value. Even *Un plus de jouir*, a "surplus-enjoyment" as Lacan would say. But it is a pleasure that is *dark*, really *dark*, if not to say perverse.

The point is that in any work – whether it be a painting by Turner, or Courbet, or Kubin, or Friederich (to name the artists among those Civitarese deals with that I personally am most fond of) – there circulates a vital energy that engages the eye of the beholder and turns it into a "gaze". By this, I mean that the work comes to life out of the profound, intimate relationship between *bios*, *psyche* and *zoe* which is enshrined in it. And always the work presents itself as intelligence about the world that involves *bios*, i.e. the conditions and ways in which life unfolds for us, the life we live, and thus the set of modalities that characterize our historical life; and at the same time *zoe*, the life that is in us, the life we live, in which the energy of the unconscious leavens, and in which our *psyche* expresses itself.

In the truly marvellous ode, astonishing in its depth, which John Keats dedicates to *Psyche*, the artist-poet manages to say all this, and the reader reads it and accepts it, together with the content of meaning that gathers in the sense of each word and the content of truth that acts in other ways; that is to say, not by addition, but by evocation, by imaginative transport, by "pathetic" apprehension.

How else should we respond to a work of art if not by opening ourselves up to its movement? It is only by letting ourselves be overwhelmed by its own "doing" – and thus succumbing to the volume of echoes and suggestions, to the interwoven drives that feed certain *works that are themselves worlds*. By which I mean, works in which the mysterious knot of world and life, of soul and senses, of eros and psyche, is leavened into words and images. Not all works are able to perform this miracle. But some are, and it is such works that Giuseppe Civitarese interrogates with erudition and devout admiration. And they respond to him; they broaden and deepen his discourse, and enrich his knowledge. And they render it more mature. And also succulent.

One comes away from reading this book feeling grateful and enlightened. One has the impression that the author knows how to make works of art speak. And one has the sensation that thanks to his openness and perceptiveness and thanks also to the "correspondence of such deep affection" he is able to bid welcome to those born to the word – those who partake with him in the analytic scene.

Nadia Fusini
September 2020

1

THE IMMINENCE OF THE OBJECT

The hypothesis I develop in this book is that the aesthetics of the sublime "tells the story" of psychic birth; that in essence it provides an allegory of the process of establishing a space of thought through the progressive differentiation of subject from object[1]. Moreover, in the art of the sublime the recurring motif of light or the window points not to a different meaning but rather to the analogous meaning of opening the mind's eye. The questions I shall be asking are: What is the essence of the sublime? Is the sublime different from the beautiful? What is the sublime in contemporary art? To try to answer these questions, I shall interpret the aesthetics of the sublime through the psychoanalytic notion of sublimation. The idea behind this is that intertwining the one with the other should enrich our understanding of both. We already have Freud's notion of the uncanny and Julia Kristeva's notion of abjection; the idea is to forge a further conceptual tool that enables us to weave together psychoanalytic theory and aesthetics.

A painting by Turner from 1837 that hangs in London's National Gallery (Fig. 1.1) offers a useful way of summarizing the basic interpretative framework I will be adopting. Inspired by the myth of Hero and Leander, the work is entitled *The Parting of Hero and Leander*. What we know about the myth is based on two letters by Ovid and the account given by Musaeus, both of which have as their source an unknown text, probably by an early Alexandrian poet predating Virgil.

During a feast held at Sestos in honour of Aphrodite, two young people fall in love at first sight and marry in secret. But they belong to different communities. Hero, a priestess of the goddess Aphrodite, lives in a temple in Sestos and Leander in Abydos, on the other side of the Hellespont. Every night Leander crosses the strait to meet his lover, guided by a lamp that Hero lights on top of a tower. One night,

DOI: 10.4324/9781003478904-1

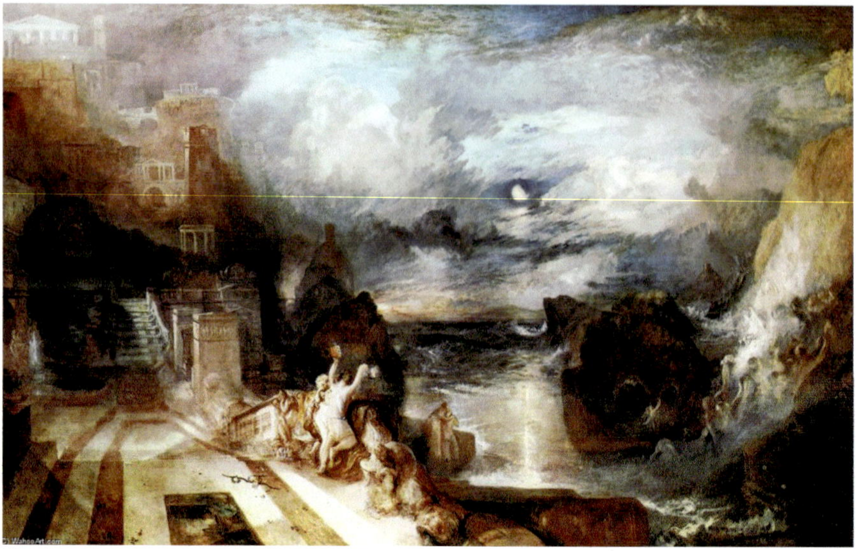

Fig. 1.1 Joseph Mallord William Turner – *The Parting of Hero and Leander* (1837), oil on canvas, 146 cm × 236 cm, The National Gallery, London

however, the lamp goes out and Leander drowns. The next day, his corpse washes up on the shore. At the sight of his dead body Hero throws herself off the tower and dies.

Before Turner, the myth recurs six times in wall paintings in Pompeii. Among the variants, the depiction found in the house known as the House of Hero and Leander, reproduced in an 1841 drawing by Giuseppe Abbate, is of particular interest. At the centre of the scene, Leander is swimming towards Hero, who is on the left, while on the right-hand side is another woman in a pensive attitude, also with her head covered and holding a lantern in her hand[2]. The image could be read as a perfect illustration of the difficult search for an optimal distance[3] from the first love object and the need to invest in new love objects. That the night crossing of the sea marks the climax of the story is not without significance. It means that finding one's way in the darkness of reality can only be achieved if someone one loves sheds some light, and that turning one's back on the object of primary care is not without mortal risk.

Curiously, in the Pompeii drawing (Pompeii, House of Hero and Leander, room z, east wall: *Hero and Leander*, ink drawing by

Giuseppe Abbate, 1841, Naples, Archivio Disegni della Soprintendenza), it is the woman holding the lamp that Leander turns away from. This detail validates a further interpretation. According to this reading, the crossing is no longer a trope of the process of subjectivation (the search for new objects to replace the maternal object), but rather it is an image of the reverse process of the return to the mother-earth and an expression of the death drive to which Freud refers. This could then be a way of reaffirming, as Freud memorably puts it, that "The finding of an object is in fact a refinding of it"[4]. Finally, the detail reminds us of the mother as the one who "dà alla luce [light]", i.e., gives birth to the infant [dà *la* luce all'infante; 'gives light to the child']. In this regard, let us turn to see how in Keats's sonnet *On a Picture of Leander*', written in 1817, the poet[5] brilliantly interprets the motif of the lamp or lantern (λύχνον[6]). He describes the splendour (*beauty bright*) of maidens, who, *Hid in the fringes of* their *eyelids white*, hold *a chasten'd light*, and who *could not see,/Untouch'd* the tragedy of Leander *Sinking away to his young spirit's night–/Sinking bewilder'd 'mid the dreary sea.* And, an instant before drowning, *arms and shoulders gleam awhile.* Throughout the poem we witness a dramatic struggle between two sets of terms, the first referring to light (*white, light, gleam*) and the second to darkness (*hid, night, dreary*), tentatively linked together by the negative principle at work in the text in the expression *not see*, two monosyllabic words that in this context only come to mean something by being together, just like light and dark.

But let us return to Turner. The left-hand side of the painting is dominated by human-made architecture and in the foreground, in the midst of various other figures painted as if they were already inhabitants of the world of shadows (and acting as a counterpoint to the spirits on the opposite side of the water), one can make out Hero (perhaps with a handmaiden by her side) holding aloft two oil lamps to guide Leander on his way. On the right, we can see a natural landscape where rocks, sea, and sky merge. In the middle, Leander's passage across the water is illuminated by the moon, but this is not enough to save him. The stormy conditions of the sea are such that the lights that should guide him are no longer shining and so he meets his tragic fate.

Thus we have a woman spectator who, complicit with the beholder outside the painting, observes a dramatic spectacle that involves her deeply. My interpretation of this is that the object that arouses in her such a passionate experience is not so much Leander – obviously, this is the case on the banal surface level of the story – but rather nature, boundless and cruel, yet also rendered beautiful by Turner's art. *By the same token, this landscape element can be seen as referring back to the object of the primary relationship.* In other words, Hero and Leander mediate the relationship between viewer and the ghost of the object depicted as infinity. As in a dizzying game of mirrors, the emotional intensity of this bond (*primary* with respect to the birth of the psyche), the erotic passion of the two lovers, and the aesthetic experience of the artistic sublime are reflected in each other.

Thus the function of the character of Leander, or rather the passion that binds him to Hero, seems equally to be to raise the emotional temperature of the scene to the highest level, as indicated by the bright contrasts of colour and line[7], far beyond what might be achieved by an element of nature bereft of human presence, however dramatic the moment may be. Moreover, his sacrifice points to the cut, the separation, the fault line in the ego that ignites the spark of thought and thus the first glimmer of subjectivity. Without symbols, there would be no subject and no object, but only an undifferentiated real. Thus, where we witness a death, what we actually also witness is a birth, the hour of birth.

The black hole at the heart of the whirlpool that swallows up Leander (the ominous, dark, elongated area that can be seen on the right of the painting) is very mysterious and intriguing. It looks like a passage leading down into the bowels of the earth. Perhaps even more directly it alludes to physical birth. In a commentary on this painting, Edoardo Albinati[8] also reads it as, among other things, an allegory of the trauma of birth; he recalls a beautiful passage from Lucretius[9] that compares the newborn child to the castaway who has escaped death and lies exhausted on the shore: "The baby, too, just like a sailor tossed/By cruel waves, lies naked on the ground,/Poor child, bereft of every means of life,/As soon as it has left its mother's womb/In throes of birth, and fills the room with squalls,/As is but meet for one who has to pass/Such ills for life".

The detail can be seen even more distinctly in Bradshaw's engraving (Fig. 1.2)[10], which is a copy of Turner's painting. The drowning Leander is a tiny figure, and it is not clear whether he is about to be spewed out from, or rather sucked into, a gigantic vortex. It is therefore impossible not to see the image as a highly effective symbolic

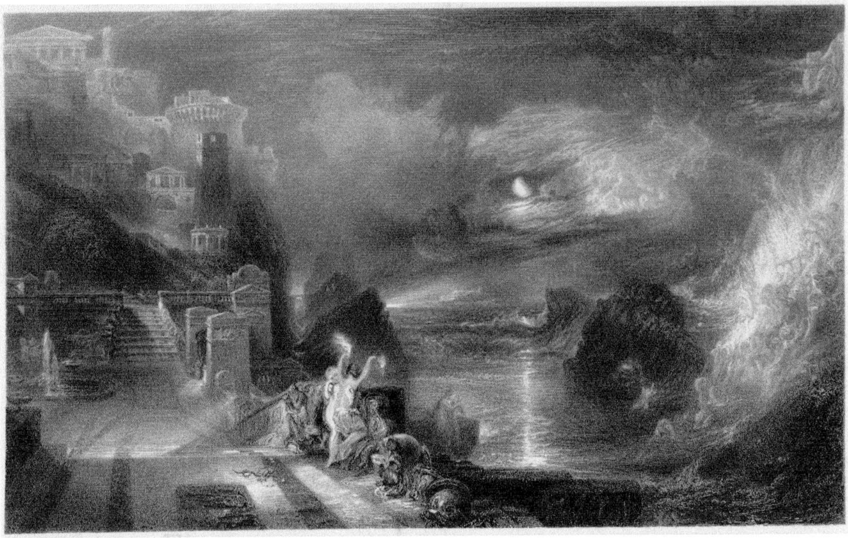

Fig. 1.2 Samuel Bradshaw, *The Parting of Hero and Leander (after Joseph Mallord William Turner),* Engraving on paper, Tate Gallery, London

representation of both childbirth and the end of life. It could be compared to Gustave Courbet's 1864 painting *La Grotte de la Loue* (Fig. 1.3), now in the National Gallery in Washington, where a tiny human figure is seen entering a cavern through a gigantic and very dark mouth.

Turner's painting also demonstrates the superficiality of interpreting the classic motif of drownings observed by onlookers as malicious pleasure at seeing others suffer[11]. The same happens in psychoanalytic clinical practice, for instance when envy or arrogance are seen merely as indications of something lacking. The relationship between bystander and the drowning person is dialectical or specular. Both are saved and both "drown". The act of drowning is nothing other than the negative upon which the self rests. Indeed, Lucretius[12] makes the point that for the spectator it is "sweet to gaze" upon someone's "troublous fate" – not because he sees him suffering but because he sees himself as having eluded that suffering. If pleasure is involved, it is the other side of the sense of security felt by those on dry land. But of course spectator and victim of drowning share the same human destiny. Life takes on more meaning the more it is mirrored in the prospect of its end. As long as there is someone to witness the horror,

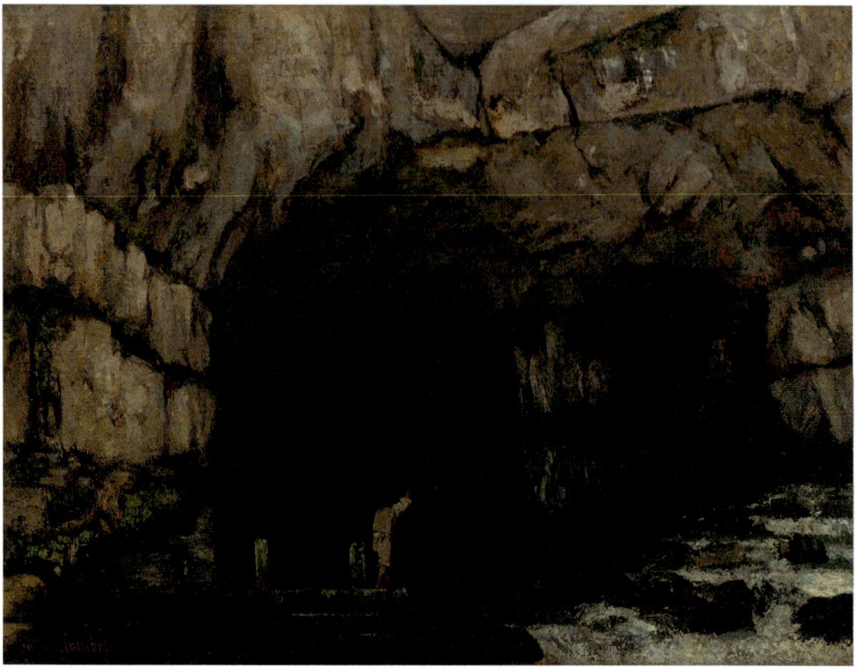

Fig. 1.3 Gustave Courbet, *La Grotte de la Loue* (1864), oil on canvas 98.4 cm × 130.4 cm, National Gallery of Art, Washington

life, or rather thinkability, still exists. The observer, not just of real drownings and storms but simply of their pictorial depictions, is not safe, he is only relatively and temporarily safe. The painting only fixes a moment in the story. Leander has *not yet* drowned and Hero has not yet committed suicide, the act she commits the next day when the sea returns her lover's corpse to her. As the Pompeian painting illustrates almost didactically, life is a crossing.

To broaden out the terms of the discourse, let us examine a few more examples of the sublime.

In recent years, Milan has seen two memorable exhibitions. The first, on Romanticism, which opened in the autumn of 2018 at the Gallerie d'Italia, gave visitors the chance to admire an 1809 painting by Giuseppe Pietro Bagetti entitled *Salita al Moncenisio* (*Ascent of Moncenisio*) (Fig. 1.4). Apart from its intrinsic value, the work is interesting because it serves as a kind of Italian manifesto for the aesthetics of the sublime. This relatively small painting depicts some men trudging up a narrow ridge to reach the summit, mere tiny figures

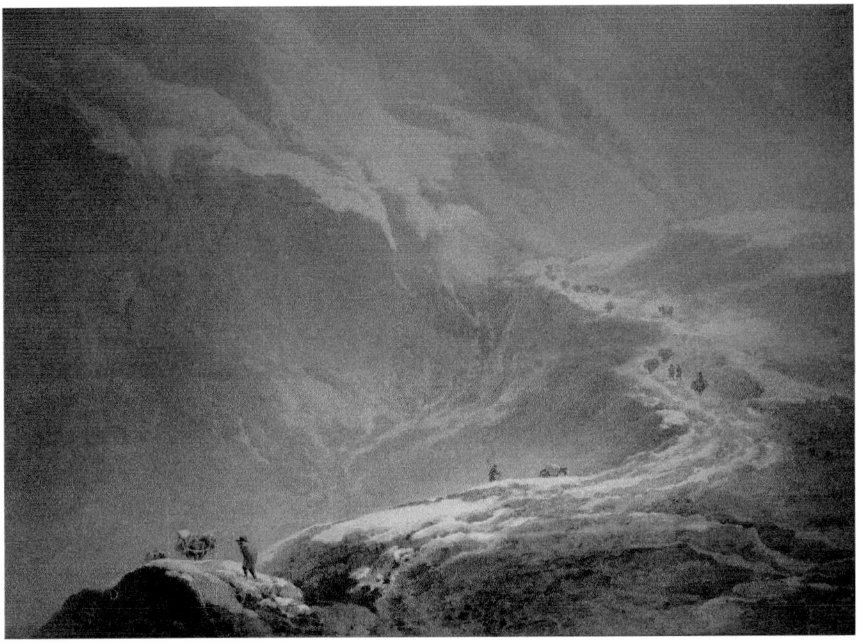

Fig. 1.4 Giuseppe Pietro Bagetti, *Salita al Moncenisio* (1809 circa), watercolour on paper, 415 mm × 550 mm. Turin, priv. coll., formerly Antonicelli coll.

against the majesty of the landscape. The mountain occupies the entire canvas and is impressive not only for its grandeur but also because it conveys a powerful sense of strength. To a large extent, the effect is due to Bagetti's decision to shroud the mountain in a mist that blurs expanses of snow with forests and rocks. What must have guided him was the idea of transfiguring Turner's marvellous sea storms into a different natural environment. As in the English painter's canvases, it is a vision that both frightens and attracts.

There's nothing automatic about letting oneself be enraptured by a terrible spectacle, because one first has to master one's fear. The necessity for this emotional precondition to be met is represented spatially in both Bagetti and Turner. While the disproportion between nature and man could not be more evident, a salvific distance is interposed between them; it is distance that allows one to control the terrible and come under the spell of its fascination.

As Sergio Vitale writes, "Pure object of contemplation, never place of contact or space to inhabit, the landscape, like his painting, is

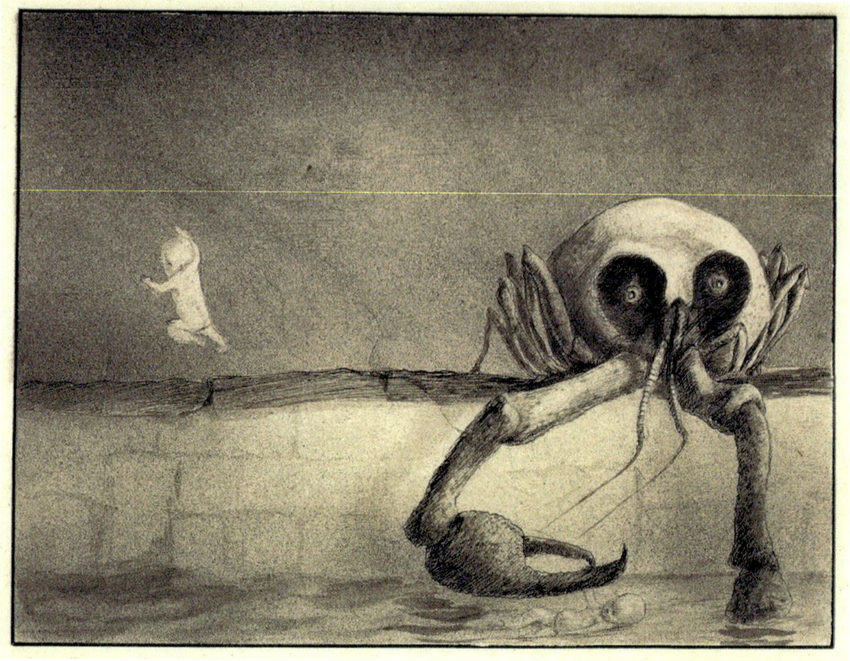

Fig. 1.5 Alfred Kubin, *Die Stunde der Geburt* [The Hour of Birth], from the Weber portfolio, (1903), 36 cm × 44.5 cm, print on paper, Leopold Museum, Vienna

born where distance reigns. It never begins with elements that are in the same space we occupy, too close and out of focus. Proximity is a harmful space that swallows up and destroys the landscape"[13].

By contrast, among the most striking works in the 2015 exhibition, *The Great Mother*[14] was a print on paper by Alfred Kubin entitled *The Hour of Birth* (Fig. 1.5). Dated 1903, it must have been conceived shortly after the publication of Freud's *Interpretation of Dreams*. On the left-hand side, strikingly similar to Leander in Turner's painting, a new-born infant hovers in the air, as if it had been hurled upwards (but there is also a suggestion it might be floating in an amniotic cavity), and has its back to an enormous hideous crustacean that occupies the entire right-hand side and is about to seize hold of the body of another newborn (or foetus) with its claw. Kubin's title suggests to the beholder a precise vantage point from which to interpret the work; however, this does not exempt the observer from asking himself what the mystery is and what the connection is between the theme of birth and the disgusting insect.

One of the most astonishing things on display at this exhibition was a reconstruction of the torture machine invented by Kafka in his 1914 short story *In the Penal Colony*. Over a period of twelve hours, needles carve out on the condemned man's back the law he has violated. When the process is over, however, the inscription written in blood is impossible to read because it is hidden behind a series of criss-crossing lines. Nonetheless, as the commander explains to the explorer, "Guilt is never to be doubted"[15]. While it is true that during the execution carried out with the cruel three-part apparatus ("bed", "designer" and "harrow"), at a certain point the condemned man begins to decipher the nature of his crime from his wounds, Kafka does not spell out what it is, and the reader is inevitably bound to conjecture that the allusion is to being born.

Now, the question is: from the perspective of psychoanalysis, is there anything these two exhibitions – and these works in particular – have in common? The answer is affirmative, as long as we allow ourselves to transpose into Kubin's child and spider, respectively, the main protagonists of the paradigmatic theme of the sublime, i.e. the relationship between the helpless spectator and the powerful and threatening element of nature he finds before him. Let us consider Bagetti's *The Ascent of Mont Cenis* in the light of Kubin's *The Hour of Birth* and Kafka's infernal machine. In other words, let us use the expressive power of one of the Palazzo Reale exhibitions to interpret the other. We could formulate the hypothesis that what these works are ultimately about, albeit in varyingly obscure ways, is nothing other than the motif of psychic birth. Or to put it another way, each enacts the emotional turbulences that colour the primary relationship between mother and infant.

One of Freud's[16] most celebrated dictums states that "*The ego is not master in its own house*". Which means that the master, so to speak, is the unconscious. That is why the analyst is always receptive to the discourse of the unconscious or, as is said, of the Other. But then Freud also adds that "the dwelling-house was a substitute for the mother's womb, the first lodging, for which in all likelihood man still longs, and in which he was safe and felt at ease"[17]. The point is that if the mother's body is the first dwelling place of being, then, on the level of phantasy, it will remain so forever, and that any future event will be inscribed within this phantasied framework. This is what happens, for example, when, as he writes elsewhere, "The field of ethics, which is so full of problems, presents us with another fact: namely that ill-luck—that is, external frustration—so greatly enhances the power of the conscience in the super-ego"[18].

In reality, at the beginning of life the primary object is constituted as the effect of an initial transposition or transference. For Freud, the object is born in hatred, but since feeling hatred for something or someone presupposes that there is already an ego, it would be more correct to say that it is born in *pain*. However improperly, it is easier to think of the infant's pain at birth as "animal" pain. Only later is pain identified with hatred for someone other than oneself.

Freud's brilliant insights lay down the coordinates for our journey. Not only a house but any landscape, for example, will never be just a landscape; unconsciously it will be identified with the maternal body[19]. Unconsciously we—the epigraph is not there anymore we transpose ourselves into all things. The line of associations then becomes dizzying, if, according to Heidegger, we remember that the "home" of being is language.

In literature, something like this is compellingly expressed by Michel Leiris[20]: "To be far away from a woman and to live in that absence, of something that has dissolved and seemingly faded away, existing no longer as a separate body but become space, the phantasmal frame through which one moves". For his part, Winnicott[21] writes that for the child the object is the emotional air he breathes in a certain environment, and that like the weather it can undergo sudden "climatic" changes.

> Some babies do not quite give up hope and they study the object and do all that is possible to see in the object some meaning that ought to be there if only it could be felt. Some babies, tantalized by this type of relative maternal failure, study the variable maternal visage in an attempt to predict the mother's mood, just exactly as we all study the weather. The baby quickly learns to make a forecast: 'Just now it is safe to forget the mother's mood and to be spontaneous, but any minute the mother's face will become fixed or her mood will dominate, and my own personal need must then be withdrawn otherwise my central self may suffer insult.

If we accept this interpretation, we can better understand why, with regard to landscape, but now understood by us as a phantasmatic substitute for the "object" in the psychoanalytic sense (usually the person who permits desire to be satisfied), Vitale insists on how important it is for the subject to attain the perspective of distance. Doing so is important because it removes the risk of excessive closeness. Paradoxical as it may seem, imprisonment in the mother's *claustrum*[22] is more dangerous than its opposite, that is to say, the situation in which the subject suffers abandonment. There is yet another reason. In order to survive, the infant needs its mother. That is why it is born in her womb and lives for a long time in her proximity, and so it passes from a material womb to a sensory womb, and then also to a womb that exists in the sphere of the ideal[23]. At birth, this closeness is guaranteed by biology.

It is a different question with distance. Not being able to gain the distance from which to view the object is a far more insidious danger. For the new subject as it forms, this seems to be the most difficult task. Vitale seems to say that while excessive distance leaves one hopeful, there is no escape from becoming caught up in a state of indifference. Indeed, as we know from clinical experience, while the first eventuality can always be remedied by a substitute object, the second, I repeat, leads directly to *Psycho*. Hitchcock's[24] film puts the seal, once and for all, on what is one of the most frightening human conditions, albeit to highly varying degrees.

In *Seminar X*, Lacan[25] asserts that the subject should fear not so much abandonment as the looming imminence of the object:

> Don't you know that it's not longing for the maternal breast that provokes anxiety, but its imminence [from *imminere* = 'to overhang']? What provokes anxiety is everything that announces to us, that lets us glimpse, that we're going to be taken back onto the lap. It is not, contrary what is said, the rhythm of the mother's alternating presence and absence. The proof of this is that the infant revels in repeating this game of presence and absence. The security of presence is the possibility of absence. The most anguishing thing for the infant is precisely the moment when the relationship upon which he's established himself, moment when the relationship upon which he's established himself, of the lack that turns into desire, is disrupted, and this relationship is most disrupted when there's no possibility of any lack, when *the mother is on his back all the while*, and especially when she's wiping his backside. This is one model of demand, of the demand that will never let up.

Lacan is only partly right because with respect to the child's needs, the imminence of the object, for example, the mother who is physically present but depressed, and who therefore does not develop a sense of trust and security in the child, is only another form of absence. He is certainly right, however, when he writes that desire is desire of the Other. It is the reason why the subject cannot do without the Other and is forced to oscillate between the risk of losing it and that of becoming entangled in it; in other words, precisely, between two forms of "absence. The balance becomes precarious in schizoid personalities in whom psychotic thinking prevails. What we see is that a particularly cruel early superego ends up preventing the mediating function that the ego takes on with respect to the needs of the id because it seems to have denied its development and even its existence.

As in certain sects, the reality principle develops imperfectly. Instead of an emotional stance of openness and hospitality, we find fanatical moralism and, as Bion[26] writes, "a lack of respect for the truth", which results in "starvation of the psyche and stunted growth". As we know, moralism tends rather to open the way for abstract and preconceived ideas which show little respect for human interest. Strict adherence to the norm comes at the expense of humanity and vitality; it leads to people living as robotic beings incapable of "feeling".

But how does a cruel early superego come to be formed? We may think that it happens to individuals for whom the experience of the no-breast[27] or absence of the breast that is at the origin of thought is not tolerable. Put another way, the rhythmic pattern of positive and negative "realisations" given by the encounter of an innate pre-conception of the breast with a concrete satisfaction, and then by the encounter of the same pre-conception with non-satisfaction is already too pervaded by the negative, that is, by painful absence. It is a "moth-eaten" object that provides truth as food for the mind[28]. If things are so irredeemable as to lead to the structuring of a psychotic personality, the severity of the superego merely reflects the hyperbolic degeneration of any frustrating "experience of no-breast" into a feeling of terror. The experience is no longer so much that of the no-breast or "no-thing", a situation in which the breast continues to be there, but rather that of nothingness (*noughtness*). The reason is that the slightest lack would be catastrophic. As Frances Tustin[29] imagines for autistic children, absence is felt as the amputation of a body part.

When this is the imprint received from the primary relationship, the child's instinctive reaction is *to stick* to the object to plug its holes. Total identification with the ruthless object, non-distance from it, drastically reduces the subject's degree of freedom from the norm, the acceptance of which is a precondition for feeling recognized and accepted, that is, for feeling that one is licensed to exist. Responses to stimuli tend to become "automatic" (as in animals). As a minimal differentiation from the object, simply existing is already a fault. As in Kafka's *The Trial*, the dominant feeling is nameless anguish ("without verdict") and a kind of passive resignation. Thus, we see that the absolute superego and any form of moralism are against life.

But we must base our reading not only on occasional juxtapositions or impromptu associations. Why else should we think of the reversibility between *The Parting of Hero and Leander* or *The Ascent of Mont Cenis* and *The Hour of Birth*? What do we make of the fact that Turner's and Bagetti's paintings can be read through the prism of the title and subject of Kubin's drawing and vice versa? And above all, what do we get out of it?

Notes

1 See J. Laplanche & J.-B. Pontalis, *The Language of Psychoanalysis*, 1967, transl. by D. Nicholson-Smith, Karnac, London, 1988, p. 273: "In correlation with the instinct: the object is the thing in respect of which and through which the instinct seeks to attain its aim (i.e. a certain type of satisfaction). It may be a person or a part-object, a real object or a phantasied one".

2 S. Miranda, "Programmazione pittorica nella decorazione parietale pompeiana: il mito di Ero e Leandro", *Rivista di studi pompeiani*, 111–118, 1991–1992.

3 When distance loses proximity to the other, it becomes laceration or mortification. See R. Mancini, *La fragilità dello Spirito. Leggere Hegel per comprendere il mondo globale*, FrancoAngeli, Milano 2019, p. 31: "Hegel's entire work can be read as an attempt to combat *Entzweiung* experienced as a disruptive separation in any form of relationship".

4 S. Freud, *Three Essays on the Theory of Sexuality*, 1905, in: *The Standard Edition of the Complete Psychological Works of Sigmund Freud 7:123-246*, p. 222.

5 J. Keats, https://popularvictorianpoetry.wordpress.com/an-anthology-of-popular-victorian-poetry/john-keatss-on-a-picture-of-leander-gem-1829/.

6 Museo, *Hero and Leander*, critical edition and Italian translation E. Malcovati, Istituto editoriale italiano, Milan 1947, p. xx. pp. 28, 30, 40. https://archive.org/details/heroandleander00musauoft/page/24/mode/2up

7 The observations made by K. Alvanson et al. ("The Real and the Sublime", *Psiche*, 1, 105–143, 2019, p. 107) about Turner's other works, such as *The Shipwreck* and *A Disaster at Sea*, could also be applied to this painting: "One scarcely needs to register the subject of the painting to experience the restless, queasy motion induced by Turner's arrangement of colour and intensity".

8 E. Albinati, "Naufragio senza spettatore", *Psiche*, 1, 2019, pp. 177–180. Still on the theme of "reversibility" between nature and humanity, in his *Mindscapes. Psiche nel paesaggio*, Raffaello Cortina, Milan 2017, V. Lingiardi quotes an evocative passage from *L'incantato* (Garzanti, Milan 1987, pp. 20–22) in which Ginevra Bompiani describes the birth of landscape as childbirth: "Then she saw from that swollen belly, on which she held her hands as she screamed, slowly emerge between her legs a soft yet firm protuberance, and then a tender brown down, and then a slight pale green declivity, and again a protuberance, more tenuous and sprinkled here and there with dimples, small inlets, and then a spot, there a clump or a clearing, and at the bottom, almost on the level of the bed, a stream of water flowing delicately like a vein. The belly had sagged and the legs now rested quietly on the sheet. Between them that green and brown yet lush form lay placidly. The young man bent down astonished. He had never seen a newborn landscape". See also S. Freud, 1900, *The Interpretation of Dreams*, transl. by J. Strachey, SE V, p. 399, The Hogarth Press, London 1981: "In some dreams of landscapes or other localities emphasis is laid in the dream itself on a convinced feeling of having been there once before. (Occurrences of '*déjà vu*' in dreams have a special meaning.) These places are invariably the genitals of the dreamer's mother; there is indeed no other place about which one can assert with such conviction that one has been there once before. [...] A large number of dreams, often accompanied by anxiety and having as their content such subjects as passing through narrow spaces or being in water, are based upon phantasies of intra-uterine life, of existence in the womb and of the act of birth".

9 Lucretius, *On the Nature of Things*, transl. R. Allison, Arthur L. Humphreys, London, 1919, Book V, vv. 222–228, p. 175. https://archive.org/details/onthenatureof00lucruoft/page/174/mode/2up?view=theater (accessed Dec. 5th, 2022)

10 https://www.tate.org.uk/art/artworks/turner-the-parting-of-hero-and-leander-engraved-by-s-bradshaw-t06350

11 See H. Blumenberg, *Shipwreck with Spectator: Paradigm of a Metaphor for Existence*, 1979, transl. by S. Rendall, MIT Press, Cambridge, MA, 1997, p. 38/VEDI IT

12 Lucretius Carus, *On the Nature of Things*, cited, Book II, vv. 3–4, p. 42. https://archive.org/details/onthenatureof00lucruoft/page/42/mode/2up?view=theater (accessed Dec. 5th, 2022).

13 S. Vitale, *Il paesaggio e il suo rovescio. Distanza e proiezione nel luogo dell'Altro*, Clinamen, Florence 2015, p. 12.
14 M. Gioni, ed., *The Great Mother: Women, Maternity, and Power in Art and Visual Culture, 1900–2015*, Skira, Milan, 2016.
15 F. Kafka, "In the Penal Colony", *The Metamorphosis, in the Penal Colony and Other Stories*, pp. 191–227, transl. by W. and E. Muir, Schocken Books, New York, 1948, p. 198.
16 S. Freud. A Difficulty in the Path of Psycho-Analysis. The Standard Edition of the Complete Psychological Works of Sigmund Freud 17:135–144, 1917, p. 143.
17 S. Freud. *Civilization and Its Discontents.* The Standard Edition of the Complete Psychological Works of Sigmund Freud 21:57–146, 1930, p. 91.
18 Cf. S. Freud. *Civilization and Its Discontents*, cited, p. 126.
19 See G. Civitarese, "Postfazione", in: F. Capello, *Città specchio. Soggettività e spazio urbano nel Primo Novecento*, pp. 187–193, FrancoAngeli, Milan, 2013.
20 M. Leiris, *Phantom Africa*, 1934, transl. by B. Hayes Edwards, Seagull Books, Calcutta, p. 237.
21 D. W. Winnicott, "Mirror Role of Mother and Family in Child Development", 1971, pp. 149–159, in: *Playing and Reality*, Routledge, London, 2009, p. 171. p. 152.
22 See D. Meltzer, *The Claustrum: An Investigation of Claustrophobic Phenomena*, 1992. Karnac, London, 2008.
23 See Isaiah 49:15 (KJV): "Can a woman forget her sucking child, that she should not have compassion on the son of her womb? Yea, they may forget, yet will I not forget thee".

W. Minella (2019, personal communication) comments: "In this passage, the nuance of expression of the verb *rahem*, 'to care, be mild, have mercy, have tender affection, have compassion, pity, affection', is worthy of note: feel compassion, pity, affection' (definition taken from the *Dictionary of Biblical Hebrew* by L. A. Schökel, San Paolo Edizioni, 2013), which corresponds to the noun *rehem*, which means 'womb' or 'maternal bowels' is worthy of note. Here the emotional, specifically visceral, foundation of compassion is very clear. Similarly in Jeremiah 31:20: "Is Ephraim [Israel by metonymy] my dear son? Is he a pleasant child? For since I spake against him, I do earnestly remember him still: therefore my bowels are troubled (*hamu me'ay*) for him; I will surely have mercy upon him (*rahem arahemennu*)". As we can see, the viscera return, but more precisely the maternal viscera, which are present in the verb *rahem*, which appears in duplicate form, expressing a strengthening of the action". The plural of *rehem* is *rahamim*, which indicates *all* wombs, or by definition *the divine womb*. Divine mercy can thus be connected to the maternal womb. This notion sheds light on Bion's and Winnicott's concepts of the capacity for reverie and primary maternal concern, respectively. But not only that: in fact we can also glimpse a link with the Husserlian concept of pre-human intersubjectivity, intersubjectivity based on instincts, on the "sexual community", or, according to Merlau-Ponty, on the "flesh [chair]". See also C. Lispector, *The Stream of Life,* p. 8. Minneapolis: University of Minnesota Press, 1989: "I slowly enter writing, just as I have entered painting. It's a world entangled with vines, syllables, sunflowers, honeysuckle, colors and words – outlining the entrance of the ancestral cavern which is the uterus of the world and from which I will be born".

24 A. Hitchcock, *Psycho*, USA, 1960.

25 J. Lacan, *Anxiety: The Seminar of Jacques Lacan, Book X* [2004], transl. By A. R. Price, Cambridge, UK, 2014, p. 53–54, my Italics.

26 W. R. Bion, *Transformations*, Karnac, London, 1965, p. 38

27 In psychoanalysis, "breast" denotes the part of the mother that the infant encounters at birth, when insufficient neurophysiological and emotional development means that it does not have the tools to bring together its various perceptions into a whole. Over time, the term also came to mean the first "partial object" and ultimately the maternal object seen primarily in its function of containing the infant's anxieties. For a more in-depth discussion, see E Bott-Spillius, *The New Dictionary of Kleinian Thought*, Routledge, London, 2011.

28 Cf. D. Anzieu, *L'épiderme nomade et la peau psychique*, Apsygée, Paris 1990, p. 58: "Psychic space and physical space are constituted as reciprocal metaphors". N. Segal comments in "Words, bodies & stones", *Journal of Romance Studies*, 6, 3, 1–18, 2006, p. 15: "The skin is the sufficient place of signification. But it matters because of the *form it holds* [...] by representing the principle of containment, it echoes our experience of being held or not being held, being complete or not being complete".

29 F. Tustin, *Autism and Childhood Psychosis*, The Hogarth Press, London, 1972.

2

A SUCCESS STORY

To start with, a bit of context. The first thing to say is that the sublime has been a success story. The inventor of the concept, the author of the short, successful treatise on rhetoric in epistolary form entitled *On the Sublime*[1] (in the original *Perì Hýpsous*), which dates to between the 2nd and 1st centuries BCE, would be proud of it. In actual fact, we do not know who the author was; he is known variously as the Anonymous of the Sublime, Dionysius, Longinus, or Pseudo-Longinus. Of incidental note is the meaning of this interesting prefix, which at one and the same time both affirms and denies the last of the hypothetical author's names, or at least situates him at a problematic juncture, given the key role played by the negative in this story. This is the mystery we would like to explore: the significance of the negative element of horror in the aesthetic experience of the sublime. The aim of the author of *The Sublime* is to teach the technique of artfully calling forth the most elevated aesthetic feeling in readers. "Elevated" and "feeling" here are synonymous with sublime and *pàthos*, respectively. As in a modern writing course, Longinus draws on a series of particularly successful examples and generously lets us in on the tricks of the trade.

The dictionary tells us that "sublime" comes from *sub* "below" and *limen* "threshold" and means "reaching just below the highest threshold"; that it is lofty, higher than any other, most noble, "sublime (in a spiritual, intellectual, aesthetic sense)". The sublime expresses "the capacity of art, in conflict with rationality, to give emotional awareness of the infinity and irresistible power of nature"[2]. Specifically, Longinus writes: "For the effect of genius is not to persuade the audience but rather to transport them out of themselves [ἔκστἄσιν]. Invariably what inspires wonder, with its power of amazing us, always

DOI: 10.4324/9781003478904-2

prevails over what is merely convincing or pleasing. For our persuasions are usually under control, while these things exercise an irresistible power and mastery, and get the better of every listener"[3].

The experience of elevation that the spectator experiences as an effect of surprise and wonder is thus accompanied by a certain fading of the thing. The idea is interesting because it calls up the analogous phenomenon that Heidegger[4] ascribes to the nature of the concept. Peculiar to every concept is its power to lift us up to the possibility of dominating the particular, but at the price of losing our grip on the concreteness of the real. We can only use the abstract concept of "tree" if we accept that we are not talking about any particular tree. And even if we are talking about a specific tree, we partly subsume it into the general concept of a tree. With numbers and geometric figures, then, the operation goes to extremes, because we are dealing with pure quantities and shapes. However, this kind of "eidetic reduction" of reality, which takes place not in the register of the visual but in the very process through which concepts are formed, allows us to think and communicate with others.

Similarly, in the paragraph on sense-certainty that opens the *Phenomenology*, Hegel qualifies as *divine* the nature of language to transcend the particular in order to rise to the universal[5]. One of the extreme consequences of this process of abstraction is that, for instance, not only do all tree species fall under the same concept of a tree, but that all objects we name become interchangeable with respect to their possible definition as "thing"[6]. Again, a general principle of the human being becomes the possibility language affords us to transpose all things. But does not Freud[7] emphasize of the object that "is most variable about an instinct and is not originally connected with it"? We can therefore say that at the basis of this interchangeability is the possibility, which must be achieved, of transposing the first object into another, of carrying out what, following Heidegger, we might call a *preliminary* "transposition".

If we pass in review the adjectives that Longinus uses to characterize the sublime, we soon realize that they may be the same as those that fit our concept of God. The sublime is pristine, extraordinary, terrible, grandiose, perfect, immense, profound, and boundless; but also terrible, frightening, shocking, and mighty. Not mere copiousness but tension, enthusiasm, force, vehemence, and violence. And yet always divine. If there is exaggeration, it is fabulous; if momentum, heroic; if passion, noble. When we then read that only a great soul, tending to pride and alien to petty thoughts, can conceive the sublime, we are confirmed in the idea that on the part of the human being it is a matter of ascending or aspiring to something divine.

In *The Future of an Illusion*, Freud[8] explains the essence of religion as the unconscious projection of aspects of parental figures onto the gods. Similarly, in the sublime, we are able to glimpse against the light the aspiration of a small and fragile self to make contact with an invincible object that looms over him. Again, with whom if not with the parental imago? Passion can also represent such an object. In the treatise, one of the examples of the sublime that lend themselves to expressing this concept are some of Sappho's verses. When she recites "At once a delicate flame runs through my limbs"[9], the poem itself can be read as describing not only the symptoms of amorous fever but, translated onto a metanarrative plane, also those of the effects that the aesthetics of the sublime are required to be able to arouse. These are effects that go beyond the persuasion obtainable by rational means; in fact, emotions (a phenomenon of "movement"), the constituent power of which is evidently felt with respect to the self.

Of course, if not containable, this power is indeed constituent but also destructive. At all events, the sublime hates mediocrity. The mediocre drags down not up. By contrast, in the sublime, the dramatic or passionate element always prevails over the merely narrative. In fact, ideally, what is required is the perfect match between the passion represented, the *what*, i.e. the content of the epic, dramatic or poetic narrative, and the *how*, i.e. the passion of language as the instrument of representation.

In the sublime, this co-occurrence is a must. With the aid of his skill in the use of language, the author transports himself onto the stage. Euripides himself, Longinus observes, "saw" "Furies and compelled the audience almost to see what he had visualized"[10]. It could be argued that the superiority of Euripides-as-author ("he had visualized") over his readers (the "almost" attenuates the illusionistic potential of the vision) lies in his ability as a sublime artist to effect transformations in hallucinosis[11]. But in general, hallucinosis (according to its definition in psychiatric semeiotics, namely, the possibility of experiencing hallucinations and at the same time criticizing them, i.e. in a situation in which the personality is preserved) is the product of the *imminence* of the object. The more the distance from the object either diminishes or expands, but in both cases unbearably, the more the subject regresses to concrete thinking in which names and psychic representations do not stand for things but *become* the things themselves.

It is a fact that the author who knows how to express the sublime himself becomes the protagonist of or witness to the events he narrates. The same happens to his readers. This dual movement of projective and introjective identification[12] has something uncanny about it. For it implies a violation of the respective frames of the worlds of fiction and reality. When it is overt, narrative specialists call this effect "metalepsis"[13]. A narrator addresses the reader directly, a character emerges from the pages of a book or a cinema screen; in certain extraordinary and austere stories by Borges, one can no longer tell whether he is inside or outside the dream; in Escher's drawings, an element belonging to the fictional world pierces the diaphragm separating it from the world of real things and ends up on the other side. But, according to Longinus, something like this already occurs whenever the reader is taken, captured, and subjugated by fiction to the point of becoming part of it. It can therefore be said that the sublime flies on the wings of that kind of metalepsis that is transference, that is, of a subterranean but continuous mechanism of transgression of narrative and ontological universes. What the rhetoric of the sublime seeks to do is to activate this transference to the greatest possible degree[14].

The problem with the word "emotion", however, is that we tend too readily to see it as a phenomenon relegated to the confines of a subject enclosed within itself. If, on the other hand, we recognize the value of emotion in laying the foundations of the self, it is because it does not remain confined to the self but goes beyond it. The subject is born and develops as such only out of the order that is generated in the dimension of intersubjectivity. In this sense, emotion – insofar as it is "shared", the result of interpersonal negotiation, and thus the vector of meaning and motivation – is more precisely a coordinated vantage point on the world, which is achieved through *ecstasy*. "Ecstasy" comes from ἔκστασις and – as befits the concept of the sublime – marks at the same time a point of maximum instability and dynamism, because it indicates my access to the other and the other's access to me, understood as a kind of divine possession (ἐνθουσιασμός) and of maximum definition or individuation of the subject, and in this respect "static" as something still, asseverated or established. It is more properly "estrangement" or constituent alienation.

Put another way, the child experiences a certain emotion depending on how it interacts with the mother. If the interaction is positive, the emotion reflects a creation of order in the body, the inscription of a pattern, a "habit", a sensitive thought, or "emotional concept". This is how the mind begins to develop even when the infant does not yet know how to use words. It is an affective logic without which there would be no abstract logic, and therefore no mathematics or physics either.

Many regards talent as something innate. According to Longinus, however, the technique for expressing the sublime can be learned. This is a way of praising culture and sociality. What else does the tendency of the sublime entail if not the ability to rise above animality that we owe to the technique of language (to something learned or τέχνη)? The sublime brings to a climax the innate human capacity for "empathy", that is, for emotional resonance with the other, which for Husserl is foundational to both pre-reflective and reflective intersubjectivity. As Longinus[15] puts it: "For the true sublime naturally elevates us: uplifted with a sense of proud exaltation, we are filled with joy and pride, as if we had ourselves produced the very thing we heard".

Reading this passage, one naturally thinks of the importance in psychic development, as Winnicott[16] explains, of letting the child experience the illusion that it creates the breast; and also of his other concept of the child's double dependence on the object, i.e. a dependence so extreme in that it occurs in the absence of awareness of the environment. In the very early stages of life, the child experiences "absolute dependence on the physical and emotional environment", and without being aware of it at all. The phrase chimes in with Longinus' observation that "Sublimity is the echo of a noble mind"[17], and "it is difficult, nay, impossible, to resist its effect"[18].

In the 18th century, it was Edmund Burke who revived the concept of the sublime. The author of *Enquiry into the Beautiful and the Sublime* launched the centuries-long discussion on this concept when he established the dichotomy between the beautiful and sublime. Soon, the sublime passed into the more specific field of philosophy and in time Kant, Schiller[19], Hegel, Schopenauer and finally, in the present day, Derrida, Lyotard[20], Žižek[21], and Han[22] addressed it. In itself, the annexation of the sublime to speculative thought raises the suspicion of an effort by reason to dominate a sphere of experience that by its very nature eludes it, dealing with an element that, to use Freud's concept, is of the order of the uncanny and doubly unspeakable, both because it is a mark of the familiar that suddenly turns horrific and because it is emotional in nature.

Thus Kant's[23] *real* contribution to the sublime lies perhaps more in the unparalleled subtlety of his discourse and abstractness of style – reading it is a kind of mystical ascent to the divine – and not so much in the content of his theses per se. The key assumption is that the feeling of the sublime arises from the moral superiority of human rationality in the face of the infinite. But bearing in mind the examples from Longinus, when faced with such an interpretation, we cannot help but feel a sense of disappointment. In both feverish and lucid drive for knowledge that characterizes Kant's writing, there is obviously no lack of brilliance and passion. There is, however, no real empathic penetration of the subject matter. From the treatise of Longinus to Derrida and Lyotard[24], the question of the sublime becomes more and more a rather sterile debate on how to distinguish it from the feeling of "simple" beauty. Where, however, the sublime lives in all its aesthetic splendour are in the painting and literature of the Romantic period. Here, the *expressive* thrust is no less than the cognitive one. With regard to painting, we need only think of Friedrich, Lessing, Schinkel, Turner; in literature, Hölderlin and Leopardi; the Gothic novel; Coleridge, Shelley, Keats, Wordsworth, Blake, and so on.

As in Bagetti's canvas, in paintings inspired by the sublime, the landscape becomes the absolute protagonist and reduces human beings to bit-players in a spectacle far greater than themselves. Storms, deep gorges, and bridges suspended over ravines, mountain peaks, scenes of undergrowth with broken trees, gloomy nights by the sea, and castles on rugged cliffs. And then we have curiously shaped clouds, almost like subliminal "inputs" that transpose the majestic and terrible element of nature into something human, given the spontaneous attitude we all have when we contemplate them to compare them to familiar figures. A geography of the infinite, or rather of the relationship between the finite and the infinite.

Less emblematic but of great suggestive power, there is also a figurative approach in Romanticism that explores the erotic. Nature depicted in the sublime is paradoxically both the most humanized there is – for example Marco Gozzi's *The Bridge of Varallo* (1818), also known as *Torrent in Valsesia* (Fig. 2.1), now in the Brera Art Gallery; how could it not evoke human forms? – and the version that, on a

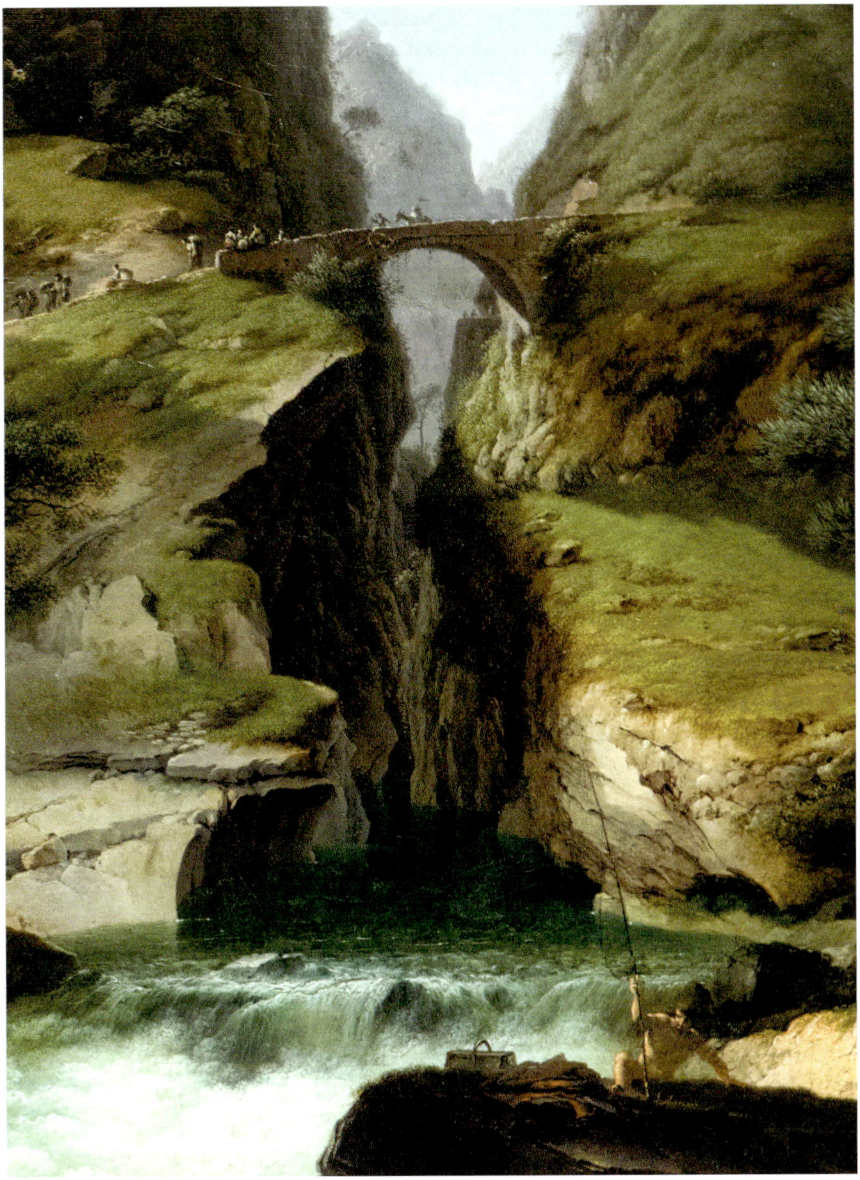

Fig. 2.1 Marco Gozzi, *The Bridge of Varallo* (1818), oil on canvas, 76 cm × 55 cm, Pinacoteca di Brera, Milan

magnified scale, seemingly best counterpoints humans caught in their fragility and limitations. The surreal element associated with it – but which is well represented by the preference accorded to landscapes illuminated by murky moonlight – is implicit rather than declared. An interpretative effort is required if it is to present itself in the light of reason. To emphasize the great and frightening power of the imagination – one need only think of the inflated and destructive role it plays in literary figures such as Shakespeare's *Othello* – we also have not infrequent landscapes of invention. Not so much views "from life" but rather landscapes of the imagination that are fictional or "scenographic".

When it comes to poetry, Leopardi's masterful rendering of the sublime in "L'Infinito" remains unsurpassed, even aside from its content, in the figure of speech of anastrophe or hyperbaton, i.e. the inversion of the usual arrangement of two or more successive words or syntagmas[25]. Repeatedly subverting the natural order of the sentence creates a sense of anxiety. The rubber band stretches and is then released. Just like Freud's *fort/da* with the spool that the grandson throws under the bed and then retrieves, thus mimicking his mother's disappearance and reappearance. But this is the very rhythm through which identity is constructed: absence/presence, no-thing/thing.

The musical phrasing of the text is such that it generates tension, yet it also helps us guess when it will end. This musical-sensory aspect functions for the reader as a *semiotic* space provided by the author, a place where the sensible and the rational are reunited. The body of the word stretches musically forward and is in perfect unison with the thrust of meaning. The "sublime" disorder of the sentences is mirrored, then, in a similar logical inversion, but in this case, it pertains to the level of content. I refer to the relationship between the two terms of the metaphor (the hedge) which comes early in the poem and leaves the reader in a state of uncertainty and the metaphorized, which reveals its meaning. It is only at this point that the reader realizes that the obstacle that materially prevents one from fully seeing the landscape refers quite simply to the end of life.

The spiritual elevation of the sublime does not therefore lie in mere reasoning, as Kant would have it. If the sublime becomes the outcome of judgment, it loses its rootedness in the sensible. Instead, the development of the ego arises from *form*, sensoriality, the body, rhythm, emotion, timing, song, and dance. I hope it is clear at this point that the stretching and release of the "rubber band" that through symbolization links words to their meanings and is inevitably rendered in the body of the word and the sentence, mirror the meeting and the parting, the approaching and the receding, the proximity to and the distance from the object. To be psychically healthy means nothing other than to situate oneself at a certain optimal and always variable distance from the object.

Notes

1 Longinus, *On the Sublime*, transl. by W. H. Fyfe, revised by D. Russell, in *Aristotle: Poetics; Longinus: On the Sublime; Demetrius: On Style*, pp. 143–307, Harvard University Press, Cambridge, MA, 1995.

2 *Treccani – Vocabolario online*: http://www.treccani.it/vocabolario/sublime/

3 Longinus, *On the Sublime*, cited, p. 163.

4 See M. Heidegger, *Pensieri–guida. Sulla nascita della metafisica, della scienza contemporanea e della tecnica moderna*, 2009, It. tr. T. Scappini, Bompiani, Milan 2014, p. 109: "in nessun luogo cresce il concetto 'albero' [...] ogni concetto è un 'mero' concetto, mai 'qualcosa di obiettivo' e quindi *solo* qualcosa di 'soggettivo', che viene a esistere nel 'soggetto' umano; da qualche parte nella testa oppure altrove, e perciò l'attività con 'concetti' e 'meri concetti' è uno smarrimento 'distante dalla realtà' senza 'vicinanza alla vita' [*eine >wirchlichkeitsferne< Verirrung ohne > Lebensnähe*] [Nowhere does the concept of 'tree' grow .... each concept is a 'mere' concept, never 'something objective' and thus *only* something 'subjective' that comes to exist in the human 'subject'; somewhere in the head or somewhere else, and thus the activity with 'concepts' and 'mere concepts' is an aberration that is 'distant from reality' and without 'closeness to life']".

5 See G. W. F. Hegel, *Phenomenology of Spirit*, transl. by A. V. Miller, Oxford University Press, Oxford, 1977, p. 66: "But if I want to help out language—which has the divine nature of directly reversing the meaning of what is said, of making it into something else, and thus not letting what is meant *get into words* at all—by *pointing out* this bit of paper, experience teaches me what the truth of sense-certainty in fact is: I point it out as a 'Here', which is a Here of other Heres, or is in its own self a 'simple togetherness of many Heres'; i.e. it is a universal. I take it up then as it is in truth, and instead of knowing something immediate I take the truth of it, or *perceive* it". This passage is found in the paragraph at the beginning of the *Phenomenology*, almost as a prologue, that discusses sense-certainty. Hegel argues that there is no perception that is not mediated by language. As we can see, it is not at all a question of the divine nature of language in the literal sense of the word, but only of its normal functions. Mostly we do not realise it, but such functions are

extraordinary. Language is 'divine' because through concepts it perceives the object and *universalises* it: "those who assert the truth and certainty of the reality of sense-objects that they should go back to the most elementary school of wisdom [...] They *mean* 'this' bit of paper on which I am writing—or rather have written—'this'; but what they mean is not what they say. If they actually wanted to *say* 'this' bit of paper which they mean, if they wanted to *say* it, then this is impossible, because the sensuous This that is meant *cannot be reached* by language, which belongs to consciousness, i.e. to that which is inherently universal" (ibid., pp. 65–66). The most authoritative and clear commentary on this page of Hegel that I know of can be read in Heidegger (*Hegel's Phenomenology of Spirit* [1980], transl. by P. Emad & K. Maly, Bloomington & Indianapolis, Indiana University Press, 1988, p. 64): "Language allows us to experience [...] what really is true according to sense-certainty. Language forces things into their opposites, sublates them, raises them to genuine truth. Language is in itself mediating; it prevents us from sinking into that which has the character of the this—that which is totally one-sided. relative. and abstract". This is why Hegel says, in the decisive closing section of the discussion on sense-certainty, that language has "the divine nature of immediately perverting the intention" [...] Language is divine because [it] detaches us from one-sidedness and allows us to state what is universal and true. [...] This furthest externalization exists only in the nearest internalization [*Erinnerung*] of language". On the divine nature of language, see also F. Cimatti, *La vita estrinseca. Dopo il linguaggio*, Orthotes, Naples-Salerno 2018: language is divine because it is 'sovereign,' "accountable to no one for its actions" (p. 22); it has an "inherently juridical nature" (p. 25); "it is a device capable of generating a potentially infinite number of different utterances" (p. 149) and through processes that are largely unconscious; finally, it is impossible to 'exit' language. As psychoanalysis knows well, no interpretation can aspire to a kind of extraterritoriality with respect to language, which is why it is itself subject to sense effects that the enunciating subject cannot control.

6 See T. Hobbes, *The English Works of Thomas Hobbes of Malmesbury*, Vol. I, John Bohn, London, 1839, p. 18: "But seeing every name has some relation to that which is named [*nominatum rem*], though that which we name be not always a thing that has a being in nature, yet it is lawful for doctrine's sake to apply the word *thing* to whatsoever we name; as if it were all one [*tanquam idem esset*] whether that thing be truly existent, or be only feigned [*sive ficta sit*]", https://archive.org/details/englishworkstho21hobbgoog/page/17/mode/2up (accessed Dec. 6th, 2022). F. Cimatti quotes this passage in his book *La vita estrinseca. Dopo il linguaggio*, cited, p. 27, which he interprets as Hobbes' affirmation of the

sovereign primacy of language over the world: "Language establishes the world of the things it names", he observes.

7 See Freud, S., Instincts and their Vicissitudes. The Standard Edition of the Complete Psychological Works of Sigmund Freud 14:109–140, 1915, p. 121.

8 S. Freud, *The Future of an Illusion*. The Standard Edition of the Complete Psychological Works of Sigmund Freud 21:1–56, 1927.

9 Longinus, *On the Sublime*, cited, p. 199. See also the translation of this same line by U. Foscolo, "Serpe la fiamma entro il mio sangue, ed ardo"; in the following lines we have "langue" and then, the last word, "esangue". http://www.fregnani.it/varia/classica/sappho_31_lp/saecula/sappho.htm

10 Longinus, *On the Sublime*, cited, p. 217.

11 In psychoanalysis, this expression points to a particular intuitiveness of the analyst, which is achieved by applying certain principles of technique, an ability to resonate as it were with the patient's "hallucinations", that is, with the phantasies that occupy his psychic reality. In essence, it means listening to any discourse as if it were the story of a dream; more precisely, it means participating fully in the realistic dimension of a given narrative regime but remembering, at a certain point, to "let oneself be surprised" even by its unconscious communicative value. On this point, see Civitarese, 2015, "Transformations in hallucinosis and the receptivity of the analyst", *International Journal of Psycho-Analysis*, 96, 1091–1116.

12 For a definition of "projective identification", see Laplanche & Pontalis, *The Language of Psychoanalysis*, cited, p. 356: "phantasied projection of split-off parts of the subject's own self – or even his whole self (not just partial bad objects) – into the interior of the mother's body, so as to injure and control the mother from within. This phantasy lies at the root of such anxieties as the fear of being imprisoned and persecuted within the mother's body; and by a reverse process, projective identification may result in introjection being experienced 'as a forceful entry from the outside into the inside, in retribution for violent projection'".

13 G. Genette, *Métalepse: De la figure à la fiction*, Seuil, Paris 2004.

14 See G. Civitarese, "Metalepsis, or the Transference Interpretation Rhetoric". 50–71, 2007, in *The Intimate Room: Theory and Technique of the Analytic Field*, Routledge, London, 2010.

15 Longinus, cited, p. 179

16 D. W. Winnicott, *Maturational Processes and the Facilitating Environment*, 1965, Karnac, London, 2007.

17 Longinus, *On the Sublime*, cited, p. 185.

18 Longinus, *On the Sublime*, cited, p. 179.

19 F. Schiller, *On the Sublime*, 1793, in *Essays*, edited by D. Dahlstrom and W. Hinderer, transl. by D. Dahlstrom, 22–44. Continuum, London 1998.

20 J.-F. Lyotard, *Lessons on the Analytic of the Sublime*, 1991, transl. by E. Rottenberg, Stanford University Press, Stanford, 1994; and "Newman: The Instant", pp. 240–249, in A. Benjamin*, ed., The Lyotard Reader*, Blackwell, Oxford, 1989, p. 245. https://vdocuments.mx/lyotard-newman-the-instant.html?page=2 (accessed Dec. 2nd, 2022).

21 S. Žižek, *The Fragile Absolute, Or, Why Is the Christian Legacy Worth Fighting For?*, cited.

22 B.-C. Han, *Saving Beauty*, transl. by D. Steuer, Polity Press, Cambridge, 2018.

23 I. Kant, *Observations on the Feeling of the Beautiful and Sublime and Other Writings*, transl. by P. Guyer, Cambridge University Press, Cambridge, 2011.

24 There are many excellent books on the history of the sublime; here I limit myself only to a basic list: G. Pinna, *Il sublime romantico. Storia di un concetto sommerso*, 2007, Centro Internazionale studi di estetica, http://www1.unipa.it/~estetica/download/Pinna.pdf; P. Shaw, *The Sublime*, Routledge, London 2006; R. Bodei, *Paesaggi sublimi. Gli uomini davanti alla natura selvaggia*, Bompiani, Milan 2008; G. Panella, *Storia del sublime. Dallo Pseudo-Longino alle poetiche della modernità*, Clinamen, Florence 2012.

25 B. M. Garavelli, *Il parlar figurato. Manualetto di figure retoriche*, Laterza, Bari 2010.

3

THE SUBLIME NOW

The sublime is not an idea that can be confined within a particular school of rhetoric associated with classical antiquity, romantic aesthetics, or any narrowly defined period of philosophical reflection. As a category of the spirit, it is constantly relevant, transcending epochs and fields of knowledge. In everyday life, we use the adjective "sublime" in connection with a wide and varied range of experiences. The word "sublime" can be used to describe a landscape or a work of art, but also a wine or, as seen in a recent advertisement that appeared in some Italian bars, a pure Arabica coffee. What might a painting by Cézanne and a dish enjoyed in a fine-dining restaurant possibly have in common? There is a quick answer to this question: the object must possess an ineffable or literally indescribable quality; literally, a quality beyond words. We use the adjective "sublime" to express the impossibility of really doing justice to something that arouses in us a feeling of both emotional and intellectual growth. Yet by definition, as we shall see, the two cannot be separated. The elevated quality in the sublime lies in experiencing a feeling that transcends the individual's ability to encompass it within herself. It is a force that pulls one towards something infinite.

Let us park this concept of *impossibility* for a moment. We will understand it better further down the line. There is one aspect of it, however, that we can discuss immediately. The feeling of the sublime implies the experience of tapping into the highest source of aesthetic pleasure. Since we are dealing with sensations, it goes without saying that they cannot be thematized. It is something we feel, something we can try to express in images – as when we say, for example, that a wine is velvety, or intense and decisive, or harmonious and enveloping. But we cannot convey our sensations to someone who has never

DOI: 10.4324/9781003478904-3

even tasted a sip of that wine. To get the impression of a true feeling, it is essential to experience it first-hand.

Another element of the sublime is *risk*. If we run through the situations that Longinus suggests are most likely to arouse the feeling of the sublime in the reader, we see that they often have to do with grand and terrible events, both natural and human. As we have seen, natural events include spectacles that remind man of his vulnerability: erupting volcanoes, vast expanses of glaciers, imposing waterfalls, and stormy seas, while in the case of the latter, it is existential events that are grand and terrible: Ajax's silence in Hades and the suicide it calls to mind; or a landscape of ruins where monuments and palaces once stood. But, as we have seen in Leopardi, if the usual grammatical order of signification is undermined, it may also quite simply be a certain sentence structure that causes bewilderment.

This heterogeneity of objects capable of arousing the feeling of the sublime is intriguing, and it immediately shifts our attention from the observed object in nature to the observing subject, or rather to the relationship between them. The common element shared by the glacier and the silence of a man who took his own life out of shame lies not in the thing itself, but in the observer of both, and in his conscious, preconscious, and unconscious capability – to use Nietzsche's[1] words – to transpose all things. When he sees himself mirrored in the object, the spectator feels a mixture of awe, reverence, wonder, and fear. But if it is true that he mirrors himself, then, as Winnicott[2] notes, what he sees is *himself* as seen by the other; whereas when the object is not responsive, the child still looks at the mirror but stops looking into it.

It would be naive, however, to think that in order for an object to awaken the feeling of the sublime it is enough for it to possess certain special characteristics. The key factor in representation, whether in words or images, is form. By bringing together these initial ideas, we can more clearly outline the framework of a possible reading of the sublime in the light of psychoanalysis. Is it not the case that the sublime reports on the process of assimilation of what is presented as foreign (*painful*) in the object through its own mediation? What else might be at work when the mother reads fairy tales to her child? Was it not Sophie, Freud's daughter, who transformed Ernst's prolonged *o-o-o-o*, when he threw the toy away, into a *fort* ("gone"), and then, when he retrieved the reel using a piece of string tied to it[3], into a *da* ("here")?

Now, the word "form" emphasizes that the process must involve the body and the emotions. The key role of passion (of πάθος) in the sublime implies that the transformation must be "aesthetic"; it must involve the body. Here again, Sappho's poetry comes to our aid. The essential element of the "subtle fire" is that it *runs* through the limbs. The absolute protagonist of these lines is in fact the erotic body. Not unlike Racine's Phaedra, when she swoons over Hippolytus[4]. At the very opposite pole to the "burning" that characterizes the sublime lies the bookish and intellectual coldness (ψυχρόν) of the false sublime.

Thus the wonder of the sublime is ultimately "bewildermen" (ἔκπληξις) under a different sign, horror transformed by form (thought) into something intensely pleasurable, danger exorcised. Examples of this are Caspar David Friedrich's painting *Wayfarer on the Sea of Fog*, 1817–1818 (Fig. 3.1), and Turner's *Snow Storm: Steam-Boat off a Harbour's Mouth*, 1842. Quite typically, the former features a human figure contemplating a distant spectacle. Adjusting the distance makes him feel *safe*.

Occasionally, as in the famous shipwreck scene in Lucretius' *On the Nature of Things*, there is someone watching the tragedy of others unfold. In short, he plays the role of the spectator. The *passivity* built into their position is another key element. Hence, we will relate it to the "impossibility" we mentioned earlier. The impossibility of expressing the experience of the sublime thus becomes a feeling of impotence to influence a sphere whose force and size overwhelm the subject.

Let us imagine that the wayfarer has either come upon the vision that absorbs all his attention or that he has turned away from it. Either way, his position in the pictorial composition allegorizes that of the beholder of the painting. Indeed, at times, they are one and the same, for example, when the subject of the painting does *not* include spectators (e.g. *Sea of Ice*, 1823–1824), or even when it doubles up, as in the case of Hero and Leander. In this case, the identification between the fragile human figure in the painting and the actual physical spectator contemplating it in the room of a museum becomes evident. This point of torsion between inside and outside is a place of vertigo. And the word vertiginous could certainly be used to describe the sensation of the sublime, as of someone who feels he is on the verge of falling but never does. It is therefore the exact point that locates the right distance from the object that frightens and fascinates. But let us try to be more precise. *What* is it that frightens and what fascinates?

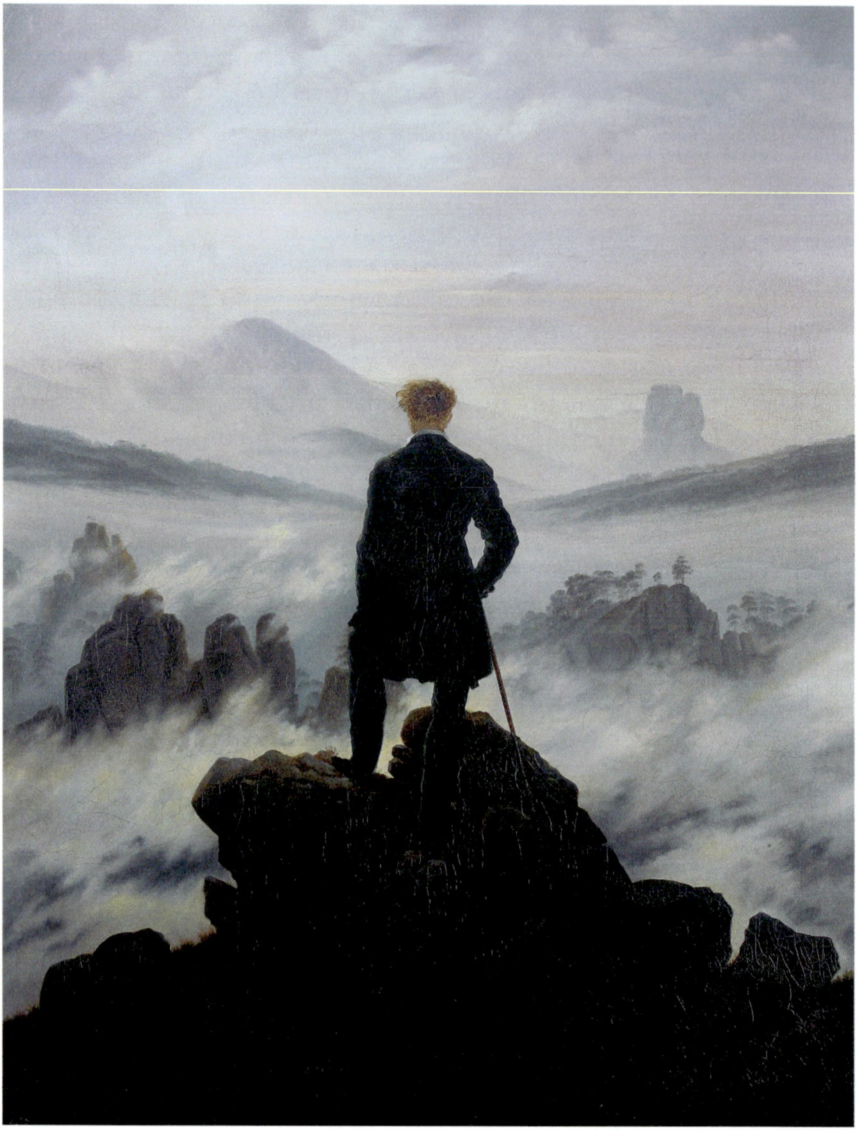

Fig. 3.1 Caspar David Friedrich, *Wanderer above the Sea of Fog* (1818), oil on canvas, 95 × 75 cm, Hamburger Kunsthalle, Hamburg

I will try to answer this question later. But for now, let us ask whether there is such a thing as a *contemporary* sublime?

The answer can only be affirmative. Not only do we find extraordinary examples of the sublime, but we discover in them a special ability to reflect their own nature and thus, by analogy, the self-reflexive essence of thought. The examples we will adduce do not merely stage the sublime. Above all, thanks to a poetics of amplification, they theorize it. In doing so, they bring to the surface aspects that remain implicit in the Romantic version because they are hidden in the μύθος. The metanarrative game sheds light on the psychological significance itself of the sublime and the controversial question of its relationship with the "simply" beautiful.

In this book, I limit myself to a few personal choices of works by contemporary artists that both amazed and touched me when I had the opportunity to contemplate them and that I regard as emblematic. I draw on my first-hand experience out of respect for the principle of somato-psychic unity that art has the extraordinary capacity to restore in us. The artists I shall be exploring are Richard Serra, Anish Kapoor, Nalini Malani, Alexander McQueen, Anselm Kiefer, and the couple Sun Yuan and Peng Yu.

Notes

1 See F. Nietzsche, "Everywhere I recognize transpositions", in *Frammenti postumi, vol. III (Estate 1872-Autunno 1873)*, It. tr. by G. Colli and C.Colli Staude, Adelphi, Milano 2005, p. 99.

2 D. W. Winnicott, *Playing and Reality*, cited.

3 See the headword "Thread" in G. Civitarese, *An Apocryphal Dictionary of Psychoanalysis*, transl. by L. Dubicka, Routledge, London, 2019, pp. 112–119.

4 See J. B. Racine, *Phaedra*, transl. by R. B. Boswell, 1999, https://www.gutenberg.org/files/1977/1977-h/1977-h.htm#linkone (accessed Dec. 2nd, 2022): "I look'd, alternately turn'd pale and blush'd / To see him, and my soul grew all distraught; / A mist obscured my vision, and my voice / Falter'd, my blood ran cold, then burn'd like fire; / Venus I felt in all my fever'd frame, / Whose fury had so many of my race / Pursued". Incest is par excellence a figure of the "imminence" (J. Lacan, *Anxiety: The Seminar of Jacques Lacan, Book X,* cited, p. 53) of the object.

4

THE SNAKE IN THE MAZE

235 tonnes of shaped steel, 20 metres long, 12 metres wide, and 4 metres high: this is *Sequence*, by Richard Serra, an enormous installation on display at the San Francisco Museum of Modern Art: two tortuous ellipses connected by an "S". By giving the work this title, in which the letter evokes both the author's initial and the form of the work, Serra seeks an effect of "onomatopoeia". In language, onomatopoeia refers to words where body (signifier) and mind (signified) come together. Serra does not do this by accident. The S, he explains in an interview, "is a passage that reverses right in the middle of the installation, and you might wonder if you are not going back in the same direction you came from, but you are not"[1].

Not that there is any lesson to be learned, he adds. What matters are the private thoughts that the work provokes. There is no pre-established path. Each person creates his or her own "sequence". The effect, observes Peter Schjeldahl[2], "is like materialised music, generated by your own movement. You clap your hands to create interesting echoes. You will enjoy seeing and hearing other people sharing the experience. Exploring these things alone, as I did, is exciting but *unnerving*. I kept feeling like an intruder in a top-secret industrial site".

Like other works by the same artist, *Sequence* (Fig. 4.1) transcends the boundaries between architecture, art, and engineering. Those who visit the installation feel the urge to enter and exit it repeatedly. The visitor feels like an inhabitant of Lilliput in the grasp of a sensual giantess, like Dr Antonio held by Anita Ekberg in Federico Fellini's[3] *The Temptations of Dr Antonio*. He walks through its spaces, corridors, cracks, retraces his steps, and then starts again moving in the opposite direction. He never gets tired of discovering new perspectives. If it is true, as it is true, that movement, kinesthesis, constitutes the canvas on which the figures of

 DOI: 10.4324/9781003478904-4

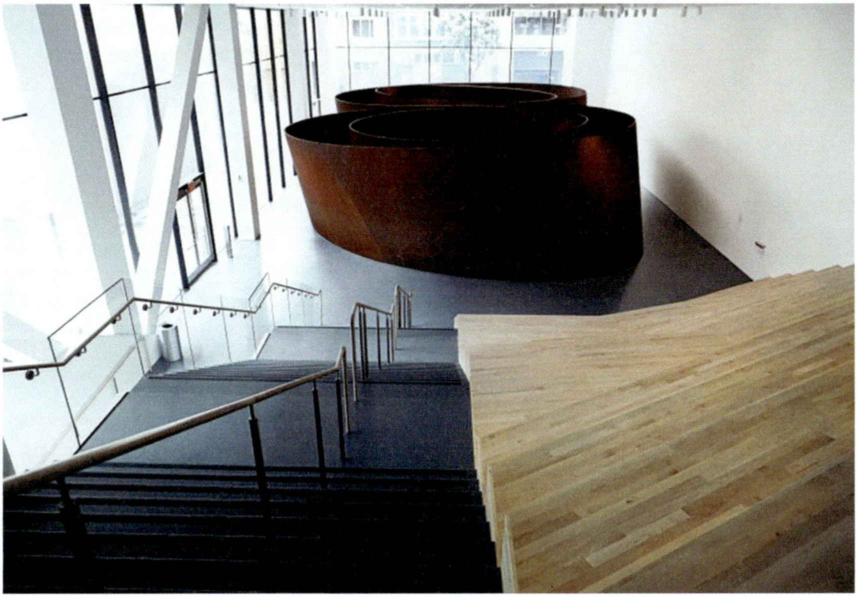

Fig. 4.1 R. Serra, *Sequence* (2006), steel sculpture, The San Francisco Museum of Modern Art, San Francisco. © 2025 Estate of Richard Serra/DACS

our perceptions and imagination are drawn, what Serra enables us to relive unconsciously are the first structurings of being starting from the state of original undifferentiation with the mother's body.

Sequence therefore is many things: cavern, door, vagina, rectum, breast, mouth, and anus. And it is also a labyrinth. One can suddenly experience the feeling of being lost. Sloping walls and narrow passages have a menacing quality. It is as if at any moment they could come crashing down on you[4]. It is not for nothing that some of his works have caused controversy and have been interpreted as aggressive, as if somehow they violated the places in which they have been placed. But the surfaces, although metallic, are warm, seductive, and smooth. After a decade or so, the steel has oxidized and turned from a burnt orange to a stable, intense amber colour. The curves are elegant, they wink at you; they suck in and entrap not only your gaze but also, in a movement you wish will never stop, your whole body.

The right distance in this case does not lie in a single moment of vertigo (or balance), but in the potentially perpetual motion that keeps one from falling, like a vortex that does not collapse as long as it keeps on spinning. The visitor is enveloped and protected and

Fig. 4.2 R. Serra, *Sequence* (2006), steel sculpture, 388.62 cm × 1240.47 cm × 1986.76 cm, SFMOMA, San Francisco. © 2025 Estate of Richard Serra/DACS

cradled, but he never knows what he will find immediately after turning: whether it will be, as in *The Cube*[5] or *The Hole*[6], the exit or rather yet another room/cell to escape from. There is no real scare, rather the tickle of a certain anxiety, the same we feel when we watch horror films, thrillers, or tragedies. The vertigo point of pleasure, what Freud calls the "heightened enjoyment"[7] that one experiences in the theatre when watching a tragedy, is sparked the instant we turn away from the pain.

A not dissimilar experience is had by those who go to the LACMA in Los Angeles, where *Band* (2006) is exhibited, or to the Guggenheim in Bilbao, where *The Matter of Time* (2005) is displayed in the main room, the Arcelor Gallery. Commissioned from Serra by the museum itself, and part of its permanent collection, it too is a monumental installation, yet it is devoid of any "monumentality"; rather, it possesses belonging, density, weight, luminosity, tension, transparency, introspection, essentiality, purity. Size is not an issue for Serra, as he has stated: "I don't think there's any such thing as too big"[8]. In fact, his sculptures are always dirtily "minimalistic", abstract, and *oversized*. *The Matter of Time* is a veritable behemoth: it weighs 1034 tonnes and has a horizontal extension of 130 metres × 24 metres. The work consists of eight steel elements bent to form ellipses and with 4.3 m high walls.

In the centre lies Snake – again the author's signature – a pre-existing 31 m long sculpture, created in 1997 for the opening of the museum.

The connection, not so hidden, between *Snake* and *Time* is obviously significant because by association it brings to mind birth the loss of Eden and the fall into finitude[9]. The sense is that the triggering of time as the subject's original temporality is certainly not innocent. In the image below, which depicts a detail of the gigantic work,

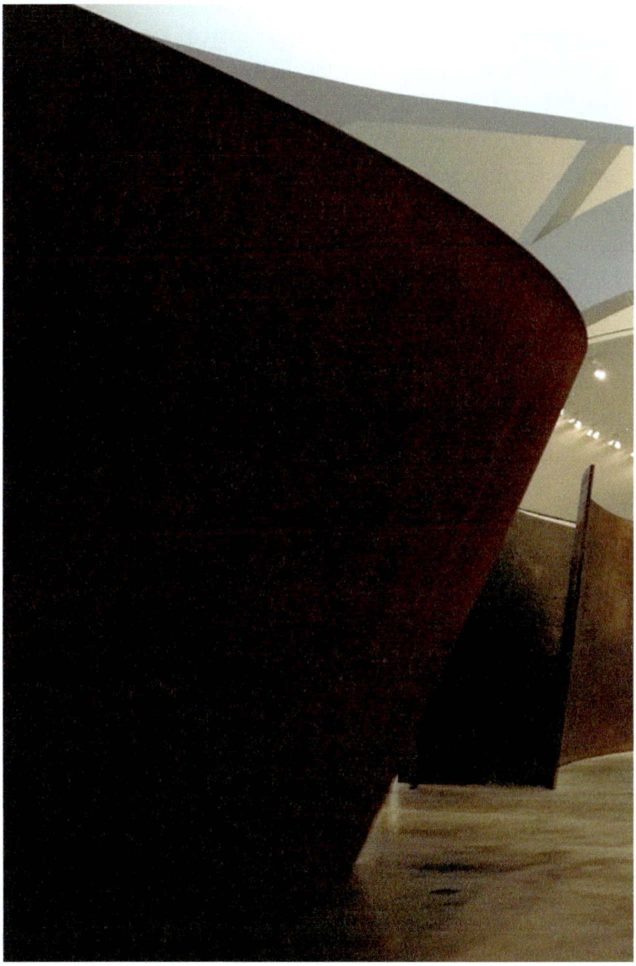

Fig. 4.3 Richard Serra – *The Matter of Time* (2005), eight steel sculptures of various sizes, Guggenheim Museum, Bilbao. © 2025 Estate of Richard Serra/DACS

caught by chance in a photograph, one can barely make out the leg and shadow of a figure of a woman or a man entering (or exiting?) it. It is a striking detail. In the comings and goings of those entering and leaving *Sequence* or *Snake*, might one not recognize an equivalent of Kubin's or Leander's infant?

The hour of birth is also the birth of the now (in Italian "ora" means both "hour" and "now"), i.e. of time[10]. But since we would not be able to not say "now" if we did not have an "I" and a language[11], we always come back to the same point: to exist means to suffer the double alienation of the inscription in the body-thing – in Lacan's terms – of the imaginary and the symbolic, that is, of a semiotic symbolic (sense patterns or habits or concepts) and a semantic symbolic (words and concepts).

Serra refuses to make figurative sculpture because he wants to avoid anything that might distract from the experience of the *here and now*. This is why he explains that he is inspired by existentialism[12]. What is essential to him is being able to rediscover the intensity of the moment. From this point of view, it might be surprising to hear him list the many different influences he has incorporated into his style, from Donatello's *Prophet Habakkuk* to Giacometti's *Cube*, from Etruscan bronze statuettes to Brancusi's *Princess X*. But it is always a question of *how* one looks. There is always the possibility of setting aside the more narrative aspect of a work so as to concentrate rather on the "force" and rhythm of volumes, solids, voids, planes, twists, curvatures, surfaces, and passages. If anyone reminds him that his works necessarily provoke associations, Serra monotonously responds with a description that reverts back to form: *Gravity* is "a square block embedded in a staircase like shape", *Tot* is "a single block impaled in the ground"[13], *Silence* is "a huge slab lying flat"[14].

If there is one aspect of language that intrigues him, it is not vocabulary but syntax. The point of syntax is to generate emotions. The syntax of the work is there to make us aware of the "syntax" of the body. This can only happen through *embodiment* and the close structuring it implies of perception and physical movement. Compared to such an experience, to contemplate a painting is, again, to move one's gaze from one point to another, thus engaging in a processuality, and yet, as in a dream, the musculature is inhibited; weight, space, and time go unnoticed, or at any rate remain in the background.

It is a paradox of Serra's art that the most absolute abstraction actually becomes flesh. Transiting from concave to convex and from convex to concave, letting oneself be guided by the curved lines of his installations thus makes sense if the mind is to resettle in the body. It is a *journey*, a keyword in Serra's lexicon, of the mind and the body. In the very act of exploring its nooks and crannies and secret pathways[15], the visitor might well imagine that he or she is the blood flowing under the skin or the foetus, coursing through the uterine canal. In his works, Serra[16] is credited with privileging not the image but the effects of the process of working with materials and the effort expended [*effects of labour*]. In our view, the term, which he uses, *labour*, is intriguing because it also means "labour pains".

Notes

1 C. Haven, "Richard Serra's mammoth 'Sequence': finally in open air and open to the public July 27", *Stanford News*, https://news.stanford.edu/news/2011/july/cantor-serra-sequence-072611.html.

2 P. Schjeldah, "Industrial Strength: A Richard Serra retrospective", *The New Yorker*, https://www.newyorker.com/magazine/2007/06/11/industrial-strength

3 F. Fellini, V. De Sica, L. Visconti, M. Monicelli, *Boccaccio '70*, Italia 1962.

4 With regard to *Gordale Scar*, by James Ward, K. Alvanson et al., "The Real and the Sublime". https://www.urbanomic.com/document/the-real-thing-the-real-and-the-sublime/ (accessed Dec. 6th, 2022), quote from J. Hutton's *A Tour to the Caves* (1781) the description of a descent to the place that is the subject of the painting. The sensations experienced through direct exploration and evoked in the painting lend themselves well to being juxtaposed with the experience of moving through the bowels of *Sequence* or *Snake*: "The idea for personal safety excited some awful sensations accompanied with a tremor. The mind is not always able to divest itself of prejudices and unpleasing associations of ideas: Reason told us that this rock could not be moved ... We stood too far under its margin to be affected by any crumbled descending fragment, and a very small one would have crushed us to atoms, if it had fallen upon us; yet in spite of reason and judgment, the same unpleasing sensations of terror ran coldly through our veins, which we should have felt, if we had looked down, though secure, from its lofty top".

5 V. Natali, *The Cube*, Canada 1997.

6 Galder Gaztelu-Urrutia, *El hoyo*, Spagna 2019.

7 S. Freud, *Beyond the Pleasure Principle*. The Standard Edition of the Complete Psychological Works of Sigmund Freud 18:1–64, 1920.

8 R. Serra, H. Foster, *Conversations about Sculpture*, Yale University Press, New Haven and London 2018, p. 243.

9 G. Agamben (*The Kingdom and the Garden*, 2019, transl. by A. Kotsko, Seagull Books, Calcutta, 2020), writes about Scotus Eriugena and his scandalous thesis that, as the chapter title states, "*Man Has Never Yet Been in Paradise*" (p. 51). The idea concerns the existence of "a most general and common nature of all things, created by one sole principle of everything" (p. 59), where the distinction between human, animal and divine is obliterated, and where sin has also always been present. The doctrine is interesting if read as an attempt to theorise in a theological key what today philosophy, psychoanalysis and neuroscience understand by pre-predictive intersubjectivity, i.e. prior to language. Not very different is Merleau-Ponty's concept of "flesh" as, according to M. Carbone ("La parola dell'àugure. Merleau-Ponty e la 'filosofia del freudismo'", *Daimon. Rivista di Filosofia*, 32, 2004, pp. 95–115) "the common ontological fabric that weaves our bodies, those of others, and the things of the world, enveloping them in a horizon of *co-belonging* in which subject and object are not yet constituted, so that each body and each thing are not given except as *difference* from the others" (p. 108). In the end, it is not that Eriugena is right as opposed to Augustine, who argues the opposite thesis, or vice versa. Each emphasises a different aspect of what humanity means. Linguistic intersubjectivity (we have been in paradise and have original sin) is an extension of non-linguistic intersubjectivity (we have never been in paradise). They are both consubstantial but also marked by a radical discontinuity. The (sublime) irony contained in such reasoning is that obviously even those who assert that man *has* been to Eden are, on the one hand, doing nothing more than allegorically pointing to a state that is not at all human but animal (language has in itself a "normative" nature; that is why being subject means being guilty), and on the other hand they are challenging our scepticism about metaphysics.

10 See G. Civitarese, "The concept of time in Bion's 'A theory of thinking'", *International Journal of Psychoanalysis*, 100:182–205, 2019.

11 See F. Cimatti, *La scimmia che si parla*, Bollati Boringhieri, Torino 2000, pp. 208–209: "The 'I' becomes something thinkable, and something to believe in, only as a consequence of the fact that we *say* 'I'. There is not first the 'I', or the mind-consciousness-of-self [...] and then the label we attach to this internal object in our mind; on the contrary, we come to *believe* that there is something real behind the word 'I' only because our language has made it completely familiar to us to speak of 'I'. We have an 'I' because we believe in language, and thus in 'I' [...] the 'I' does not exist as an entity in itself'". And further, p. 225: "'*Our* time, and in particular the feeling that it forms a unified, linear fabric, depends on language'".

12 R. Serra, H. Foster, *Conversations about Sculpture*, cited, p. 255: "Basically my grounding is in existentialism: it's the will within the moment, drawing on the intensity of that moment, that makes the difference".
13 Serra, Foster, *Conversations about Sculpture*, cited, p. 153.
14 Serra, Foster, *Conversations about Sculpture*, cited, p. 158.
15 Looking back at the formative period he spent in Italy, Serra tells of his interest in human anatomy: "In the Museo della Specola in Florence there are stuffed cadavers by Clemente Susini made of wax, slit from scrotum to throat, and opened up so you can see the splayed intestines. They're extraordinarily beautiful and also perverse and sexual. Nancy Graves and I (we were together then) used to go look at them" (Serra, Foster, *Conversations about Sculpture*, p. 16).
16 Serra, Foster, *Conversations about Sculpture*, p. 179.

5

A SPACE FULL OF DARKNESS

On 13 August 2018, newspapers reported an incident that had occurred at the Fundação de Serralves, Porto's Museum of Contemporary Art: a 60-year-old Italian visitor had fallen into an installation by Anish Kapoor. Inspired by a painting by Andrea Mantegna, the work was called *Descent Into Limbo* (Fig. 5.1) – a clear invitation to a more… immersive experience!

Created in 1992 for *Documenta* (9), it consisted of a cube-shaped concrete building with each side measuring 6 metres. Inside, there was a hole (or "well") in the middle of the floor, fortunately only 2 metres deep and 2.5 metres in diameter. The work was part of the exhibition *Anish Kapoor: Works, Thoughts, Experiments*. The sculpture, it was said, was an expression of Kapoor's interest in the formal and metaphorical interplay between light and dark, outside and inside, finite and infinite. The museum's director, Fernando Rodrigues Pereira, then declared that all safety protocols had been followed, the man had not suffered any serious consequences and had been released after a brief stay in hospital, but that nevertheless the installation would remain temporarily closed for a while.

It could be read on the artist's website that this was not a "hole" in the floor or a *"pit covered in black paint"*, as the newspapers had described it, but rather a "space full of darkness". The intention was to create the optical illusion of an infinite void or a circle painted black. The effect would have been even more effective if Kapoor had at the time already been able to use Vantablack, the paint manufactured by Surrey NanoSystems, to which he secured the exclusive rights, and which delivers the blackest blackness there is. Just like the strange astronomical formations known as black holes, Vantablack almost swallows up the light that hits it. "Just imagine", Katharine Schwab[1]

 DOI: 10.4324/9781003478904-5

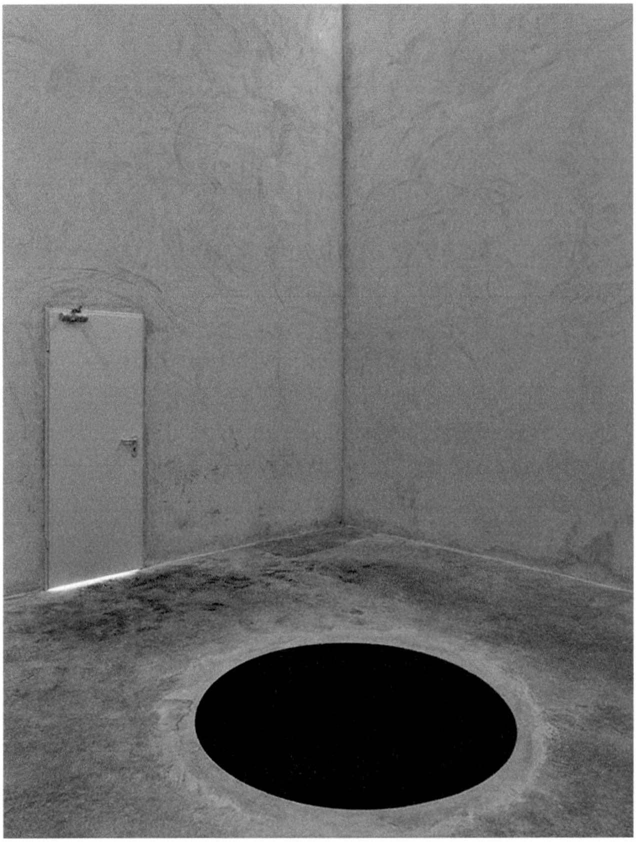

Fig. 5.1 Anish Kapoor, *Descent into Limbo* (1992), Fundação de Serralves, Porto 2018[2]

comments wryly, "how many more wayward visitors would end up at the bottom if the pit was made with Vantablack, instead".

This curious incident inadvertently demonstrates what can happen when the moment of vertigo actually produces a fall. The height of irony (the truly sublime) is that it could just as well have been preordained and been part of a performance (including admission to hospital). In terms of phantasy, the spectator did not fall into a shallow pit painted black, but into the void, into *infinity*. The dark object of desire exerted its fatal attraction. No counterforce triggered by the feeling of being confronted by something abject was able to offset its force. The threat of the imminence of the object took effect – a more

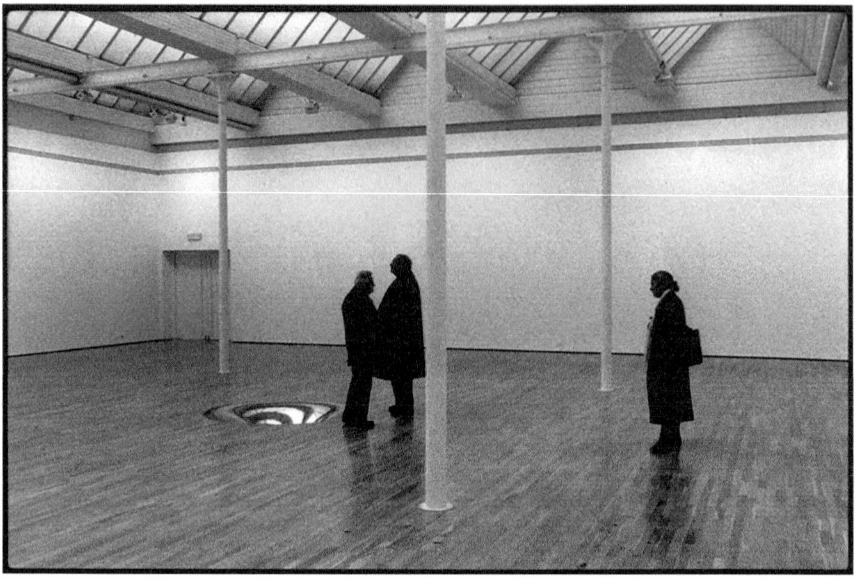

Fig. 5.2 Anish Kapoor, *Turning the World Inside Out II* (1995), 180 cm × 180 cm × 130 cm, Fondazione Prada, Milan

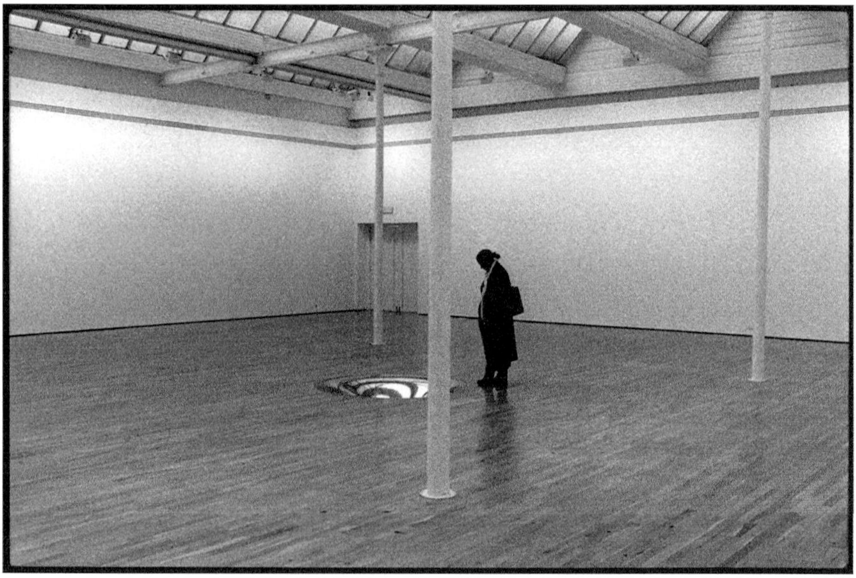

Fig. 5.3 Anish Kapoor, *Turning the World Inside Out II* (1995), 180 cm × 180 cm × 130 cm, Fondazione Prada, Milan

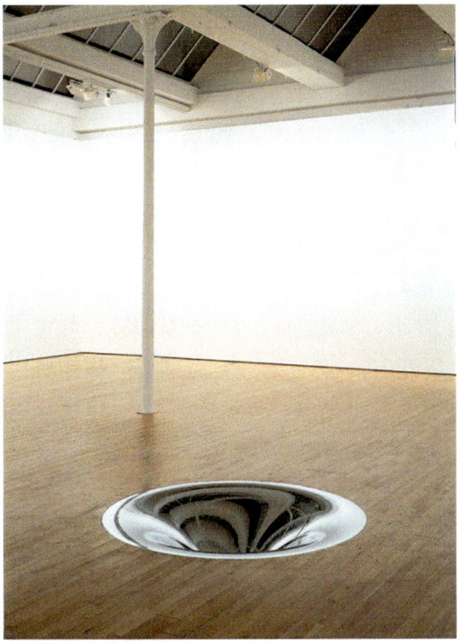

Fig. 5.4 Anish Kapoor, *Turning the World Inside Out II* (1995), 180 cm × 180 cm × 130 cm, Fondazione Prada, Milan

serious threat than that of abandonment. Not only did the "shadow of the object [fall] upon the ego", as Freud[3] says of those whose state of depression leads them to reproach themselves for absurd things (while in reality, they are blaming the mother with whom they unconsciously identify), but the ego sank *materially* at that point.

Like Serra, in so many of his works Kapoor generates in the viewer a sense of the sublime not only through the enigmatic and, as we have seen, through the unintentional and concrete dangerousness of the object, but also through its size. This was the case for *Symphony for a Beloved Sun*, an exhibition held in 2013 at the Martin-Gropius-Bau in Berlin which consisted of various works dating from 1979 onwards and a previously unseen installation set up in the museum's atrium. The title of the exhibition was inspired by the Futurist work *Victory over the Sun*, 1913, by Velimir Khlebnikov, Kasimir Malevich, and Mikhail Matyushin, whose famous poster designed by El Lissitsky is invoked. The introductory essay by Norman Rosenthal, the curator of the exhibition, quotes a verse from Ezekiel 32:6 in its epigraph: "I will drench the land with your flowing blood all the way to the mountains"[4].

It is difficult to imagine a more powerful symbolic concentration than that achieved by setting together the images of the sun and blood. And again, the cover to the catalogue of *Symphony for a Beloved Sun* features a red spot against a pale-yellow background, a blood-coloured sun. As if it had fallen there by mistake, it then reappears in the following pages superimposed over the typographic characters, even in the front matter, gradually reducing in size until it finally disappears on page 10.

Not only that. How can we not think that beloved (\bi-'ləvd) sounds almost like *blood* (\'bləd)? A text that literally "bleeds" from its wounds. So a sun, but a blood-coloured sun. It is no coincidence that Rosenthal then quotes a poem from Baudelaire's[5] *The Flowers of Evil*, "The Fountain of Blood": "It seems to me at times my blood flows out in waves/Like a fountain that gushes in rhythmical sobs./I hear it clearly, escaping with long murmurs,/But I feel my body in vain to find the wound./Across the city, as in a tournament field,/It courses, making islands of the paving stones,/Satisfying the thirst of every creature/And turning the color of all nature to red./.../But love is to me only a bed of needles/Made to slake the thirst of those cruel prostitutes!". In this poem, and generally in the *Fleurs*, in rhythm, tone, and imagery, Baudelaire uses the lofty style of the sublime but for subjects that are not "elevated"[6]. The same can be said for Kubin and his terrible spider.

Among the main themes of the poem, which Rosenthal evidently summons up in order to suggest an interpretation that is in tune with the one we are trying to outline here: the failure to recognize love symbolized by the "bed of needles", that which produced the wound from which the blood gushes; and, most notably in the context of our discourse, the fact that the violent feeling of pain (the blood gushes "in spurts" as from a "fountain") tinges the *whole* world with itself.

The haemorrhage is therefore not concrete, but a kind of internal haemorrhagic shock; as when, in the words of Wilfred R. Bion, one "bleeds" into one's own tissues, but out of a lack of emotions[7].

> Paradoxically this explosion is so violent and is accompanied by such immense fear—hereafter referred to as psychotic fear or psychotic panic—that the patient may express it by sudden and complete silence (as if to go to an extreme as far from a devastating explosion as possible). The ensuing state can be most easily

expressed by using surgical shock as a model: in this the dilatation of the capillaries throughout the body so increases the space in which blood can circulate that the patient may bleed to death in his own tissues. Mental space is so vast compared with any realization of three-dimensional space that the patient's capacity for emotion is felt to be lost because emotion itself is felt to drain away and be lost in the immensity.

How can we not think of Jean Laplanche's theory of the unconscious as created in the child by the remnants of enigmatic sexual messages sent by the mother? But even before that, how can we not be reminded of Melanie Klein's descriptions of the mother's body as a phantasmatic space that the child obsessively explores? Perhaps even more than in Kapoor's works – but with the important exception, as we shall see, of *Leviathan* – this aspect is most striking in Serra's. Indeed, in addition to contemplating the work with it in front of one's eyes, like Alice in a mirror, one can actually enter into it – even though the three-dimensional spatiality of Kapoor's sculptures invariably summons up the environment that receives them where they are situated to participate as a protagonist in the installation, certainly not as a mere container; and indeed, it always sets up a challenge between container and content.

Over time the experimentation with colour we find in Kapoor's work has increasingly honed in on red, as in the wax piles that are part of the installation *Symphony for a Beloved Sun* located in the museum's central atrium. Elevator belts incessantly transport pieces of it upwards, and then let them plummet down like spills of blood. These fragments of matter, Rosenthal[8] writes, suggest the idea of a disaster that has already occurred. Another association he makes is with Oswald, the character in Ibsen's *Spectres* who, dying of syphilis, beseeches "Mother, give me the sun". As one does when we are dealing with the dispersed elements of a dream or a rebus, it is difficult to resist the temptation to recompose *beloved/sun*, *blood/son*, and *mother* in the myth of the object that petrifies or kills. One also thinks of Medea, a character we will find in Nalini Malani, and of Julia Kristeva's concept of abjection.

Many of the titles of works in the exhibition evoke the theme of the body and birth: *Wound*, *The Earth*, *L'origine du monde*, *My Body your Body*, *When I am Pregnant*, *Organ*, *Memory*, *Negative Box Shadow*, *Her Blood*, *Hexagon Mirror*, *Non-Object*, *Vertigo*, *C-Curve*, *Sky Mirror*,

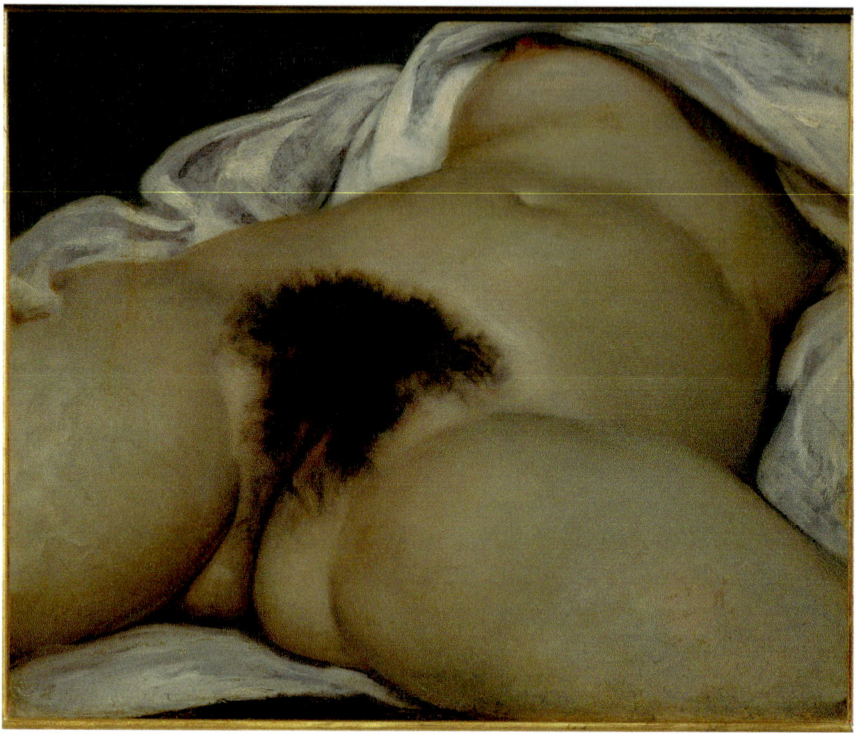

Fig. 5.5 Gustave Courbet, *L'origine du monde* [The Origin of the World] (1866), oil on canvas, 46 cm × 55 cm, Musée d'Orsay, Paris

Red, *Blood Mirror IV*, *Dismemberment of Jeanne d'Arc*, *1st Body*. But in the artificial sequence of the layout devised by the curator of the catalogue (and yet "timely" if we refer to it in terms of respecting the strictly chronological order according to which they were conceived), even more significant become the many *Untitled* works on the list. It is as if their function is to allude to a dramatic oscillation between something that can be given a name and something that is nameless and therefore frightening ("*nameless dread*"[9]).

Intermediate terms between the *Untitled* works and the explicitly titled *L'origine du monde* as a clear reference to Courbet's scandalous 1866 painting, owned for a time by Lacan[10], in which a vagina is in full view, are the various *Dirty Corner*, *Black Matter*, *Black Fire*, *Shooting into the Corner*, *Mars*, *Fragment I*, *Fragment II*, *Matt Black*, *Spittle*, *Splush*, *Splodge*, *Splat*. More than in other works, what the *Untitled* works show are cracks, holes, windows, pertuos, passages, ducts, openings, and more often than not an impenetrable deep blackness.

It is suggestively relevant to our discourse that, in terms of subject and composition, Courbet's painting is "anticipated" by Kubin's equally scandalous drawing *Death Leap* (*Der Todessprung*), from 1901 to 1902, in other words, from the same year as *The Hour of Birth*, and is followed by Rosemarie Trockel's "updated" version, *Replace Me*, from 2011. In this umpteenth variation on the theme, as if interpreting the two drawings, but brought up to date in Courbet's painting, a huge and repugnant spider is now stuck to the naked female genitals.

But it is through *Leviathan* (2011) and *The Death of the Leviathan* (2011–2013) that the dimensional brand of the sublime, what Kant calls the "mathematical" sublime, becomes striking. The immense curved forms of *Leviathan* (38 m high, 100 m long, and 70 m wide) cannot but recall Serra's *Sequence*, *Band*, and *The Matter of Time* and the beautiful and terrible – or, bringing in again the Freudian concept of the uncanny, the familiar and the alien – forms of the object. Serra, then, not only like Kapoor, goes beyond the caesura between sculpture and architecture, but also between the organic

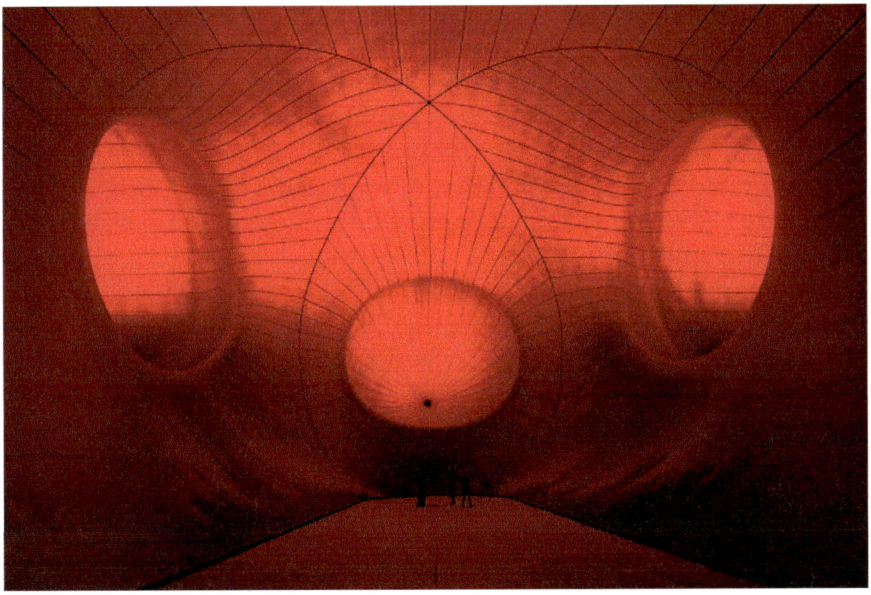

Fig. 5.6 Anish Kapoor, *Leviathan*, 33.5 m × 100 m × 72 m, Grand Palais, Paris 2011[11]

and the inorganic. Inspired by references to the *Bible* and Hobbes, Leviathan is the figure of a grandiose and destructive – yet also magnetic – power. Hors Bredekamp, who writes about it in the catalogue, references Cassandra; as we shall see, this is the other mythological figure that returns in Nalini Malani's *In Search of the Vanished Blood*.

In an interview he gave on the occasion of the inaugural exhibition at the Grand Palais in Paris in 2011, Kapoor[12] emphasizes that his intention with *Leviathan* was not so much to produce a story but to arouse a certain sensibility, and he references Hobbes, who uses the figure of Leviathan to indicate the monster-state, but also "a monster with an oversized body, which cannot be controlled, a kind of formless and primitive matter". He goes on to explain that if he sought a particular shade of dark red like blood, it was meant to ensure that upon entering *Leviathan*, the visitor has the impression of being in a space that resembles the inside of a body. He is thus able to completely reverse the perspective from which he looks at himself, the viewpoint of being able to see the diaphanous membrane of his own skin from the other side, but also from the *other* side of himself – *it might as well be the body and skin of a stranger.* He not only sees but also *becomes* the blood, flowing under the skin – an organic liquid but above all a vital essence. The more familiar vision of feeling contained by the skin is thus reversed into the perturbing one of feeling alienated from it. It is no wonder then that, like a powerful magnet, the vision attracts one's attention. It is like being sucked into a "visceral" space, in both the strict and derived sense – that is, both material and virtual at the same time – where each can continually negotiate the possibility of being alive and vital.

In the individual, the traumas that halt this process of continuity of being (*going on being*) generate an anxiety of annihilation that Winnicott[13] likens to the state, described by Ernst Jones, of "aphanisis" or disappearance of the *libido*. The occurrence of such a condition would cause a deeper anguish than the castration complex. Lacan reinterprets it as the "normal" disappearance (*fading away*) of the subject from the network of signifiers, none of which in itself could ever fully account for the subject's being. What Winnicott means, then, is the dramatic impossibility of any referral from one to the other of the links in this chain: like jumping but not finding a new foothold and thus falling into the void.

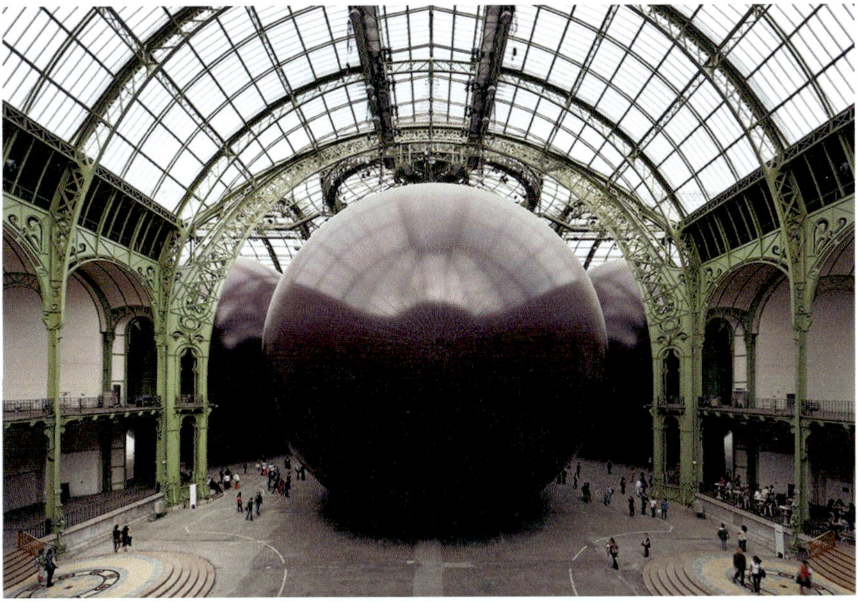

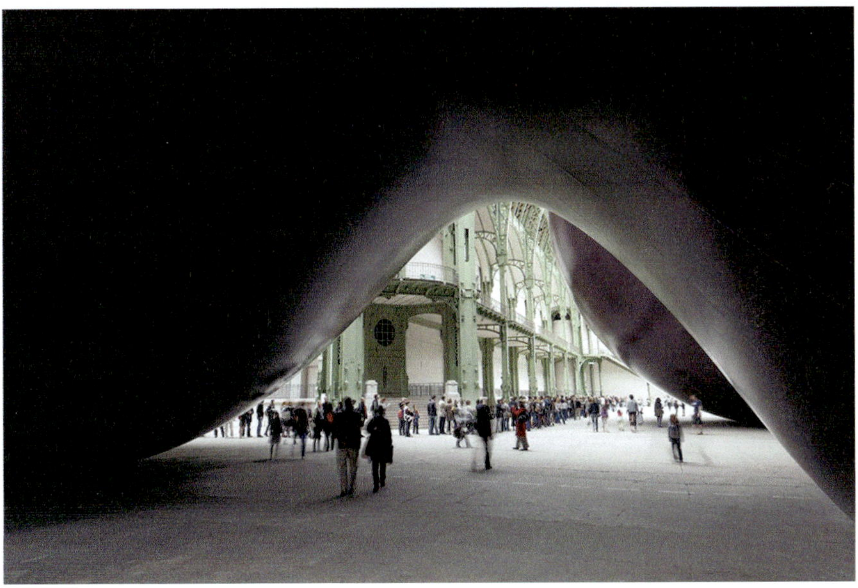

Fig. 5.7 Anish Kapoor, *Leviathan*, 33.5 m × 100 m × 72 m, Grand Palais, Paris 2011

Notes

1 K. Schwab, "Someone fell into artist Anish Kapoor's bottomless pit sculpture", https://www.fastcompany.com/90222287/someone-fell-into-artist-anish-kapoors-black-hole-installation

2 https://www.mirror.co.uk/interactives/anish-kapoors-super-black-artwork-13116313

3 S. Freud, Mourning and Melancholia. The Standard Edition of the Complete Psychological Works of Sigmund Freud 14:237–258, 1917, p. 249.

4 N. Rosenthal, "Anish Kapoor. The Artist in the Echo Chamber", 9–27, in A. Kapoor, *Symphony for a Beloved Sun*, edited by N. Rosenthal, Verlag der Buchhandlung Walther Kønig, Koln 2013, p. 9.

5 https://www.poetryverse.com/charles-baudelaire-poems/the-fountain-of-blood

6 See also E. Auerbach, "The Aesthetic Dignity of the 'Fleurs Du Mal'", transl. by R. Manheim, in *Scenes from the Drama of European Literature*, 201–226, University of Minnesota Press, Minneapolis, 1984.

7 W. R. Bion, *Attention and Interpretation*, 1970, Karnac, London, p. 12.

8 See D. W. Winnicott, "Fear of Breakdown", 1963?, in *Psycho-Analytic Explorations*, pp. 87–95, Routledge, London, 1989.

9 In *Learning from Experience*, 1962, Heinemann, London 1962, p. 96, W. R. Bion describes an emotional situation in which the infant feels the fear of dying, only to split this feeling off from itself and project it into the womb "together with envy and hatred for the undisturbed". If the mother is unable to transform the infant's anguish and allow it to "re-introject a now tolerable and consequently growth-stimulating part of its personality […] The infant who started with a fear he was dying ends up by containing a nameless dread".

10 On this painting, see S. Žižek, 2000, *The Fragile Absolute: Or, Why Is the Christian Legacy Worth Fighting For?*, cited, p. 37: "the exposed female body is the impossible object which, precisely because it is unrepresentable, functions as the ultimate horizon of representation whose disclosure is forever postponed – in short, as the Lacanian incestuous Thing. Its absence, the Void of the Thing, is then filled in by 'sublimated' images of beautiful but not totally exposed female bodies – by bodies which always maintain a minimal distance towards *That*".

11 https://de.phaidon.com/agenda/art/picture-galleries/2011/may/31/inside-the-belly-of-the-monster-anish-kapoors-leviathan/

12 C. Ecoffet, "Interview with Anish Kapoor", *Monumenta* 2011, Grand Palais, Paris https://www.youtube.com/watch?v=12Ni0c4D27Y (accessed Aug 24th, 2019).

13 D. W. Winnicott, *Maturational Processes and the Facilitating Environment*, cited, p. 41.

6

THE RIVER-GOD OF BLOOD

Speaking in an interview, the prolific socially engaged artist, Nalini Malani[1] declared her love for Italian painting, naming artists such as Piero della Francesca, Giotto, Fra Angelico, and Masaccio, as well as dor Francis Bacon and Hieronymus Bosch. She also admitted to having some familiarity with the theories of Sigmund Freud, Karl Abraham, Melanie Klein, Wilfred R. Bion, Betty Josephs, and Hanna Segal.

The work of hers I will focus on here is the installation presented at *Documenta* (13), the 2012 edition of the international art exhibition in Kassel, entitled *In Search of the Vanished Blood*, inspired by Christa Wolf's[2] novel *Cassandra* and by R.M. Rilke's *The Notebooks of Malte Laurids Brigge*[3]. The soundtrack to the work consisted of a collage of quotations from Heiner Müller's[4] *Die Hamletmaschine*, Samuel Beckett's[5] *Krapp's Last Tape*, and Mahasweta Devi's[6] *Draupadi*. The title is taken from the Urdu poem *Lahu Ka Surag*.

The use of these varied materials gives an idea of the dizzying intertextual play that distinguishes this work. And yet, the more explicit references one comes across, the more one realizes that while they have indeed been essential to the work of this artist as a brilliant *bricoleur*[7], it can well do without them and they have now been transfigured into something totally different. We will see something similar later on when we look at Anselm Kiefer's *The Heavenly Palaces*. On the other hand, this accumulation contrasts with the extreme work of subtraction or "destruction" that lies behind Serra's and Kapoor's installations.

Visitors to *In Search of the Vanished Blood* (Fig. 6.1) enter a large circular room that is immersed in semi-darkness where they are exposed to intense sensory, visual, acoustic, and kinesthetic stimulation.

DOI: 10.4324/9781003478904-6

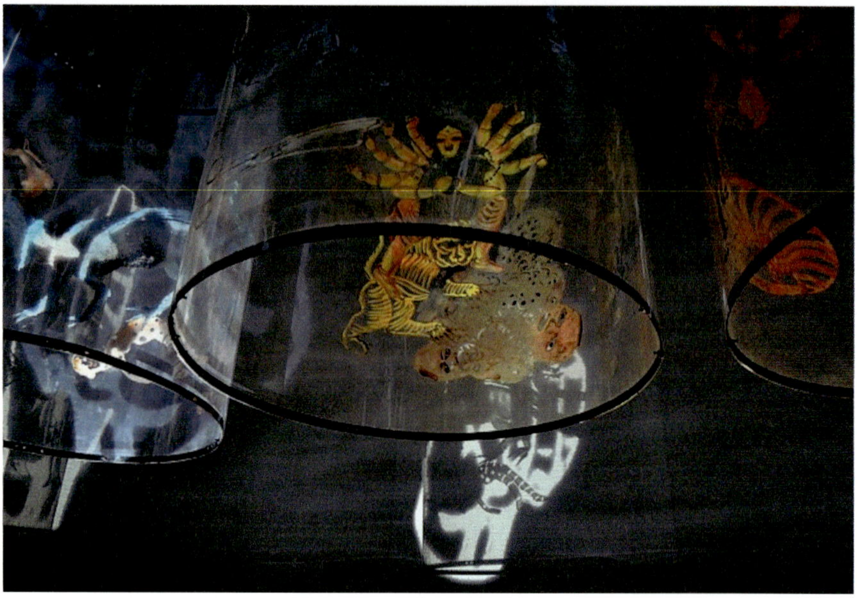

Fig. 6.1 Nalini Malani, *In Search of the Vanished Blood*, *Documenta* (13), Kassel 2012

As they move through the installation, they contemplate a play of shadows that, almost in an allusion to the psychic mechanism Freud describes as being at work in traumatic dreams, obeys a sort of demonic repetition compulsion. In effect, what Malani has organized by setting up her extraordinary stage machine is an intensely dreamlike space, where the spectator can never grasp everything at a glance. It is a way of alluding to the presence of the unconscious and the narrowness of consciousness, to the visible made invisible and vice versa.

Occupying the centre of the room are five cylinders suspended from the ceiling. On their translucent surfaces are mythological figures, monsters, and scenes from mystery rites. In powerful beams of light, projectors fixed to the walls transmit images that intercept the ever-changing images of the cylinders, hybridize with them and generate surprising effects on the opposite walls. These combine to form a single circular screen that completely envelops the spectator. *Wunderkammer*, diorama, whale's belly, Pandora's box, amniotic cavity, vortex of the Maelstrom, interior of the maternal body as described in Melanie Klein – it is an interiority that unceasingly extrudes itself outwards.

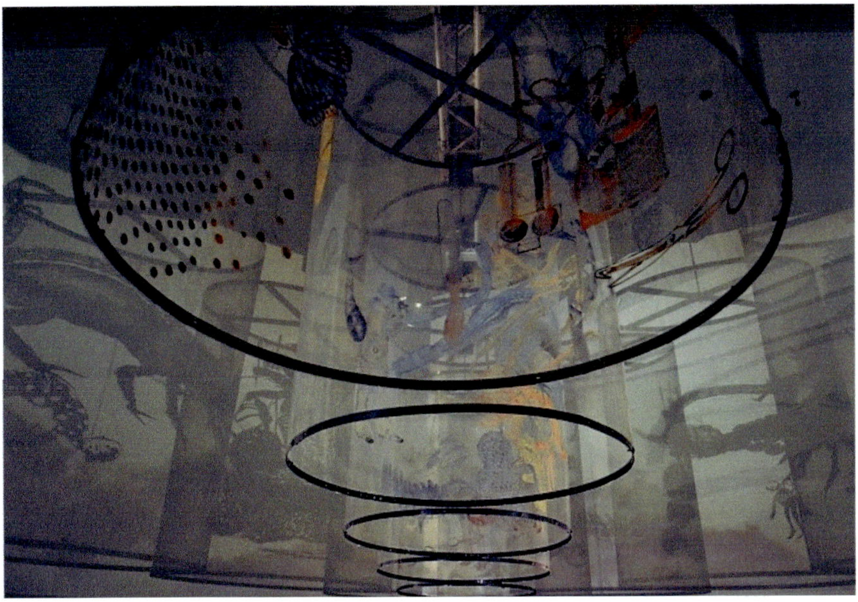

Fig. 6.2 Nalini Malani, *In Search of the Vanished Blood,* Documenta (13), Kassel 2012

All around are images of bizarre objects, mysterious animals, unreal landscapes, ruthless cruel rituals, and anatomical details of the human body. They resemble the phantasms we encounter in dreams and even more so in nightmares. Monsters, blood, horror, perhaps human sacrifices. As in *Apocalypse Now*[8], each visitor becomes a Marlowe inexorably attracted by the allure of Kurtz's magnetic fluid. Ultimately, the central theme is blood, the same blood we will see later on the mannequins in the Alexander McQueen exhibition catalogue. Anxiety, enchanted wonder, religious awe, and curiosity chase one another along with a sense of bemusement and excitement.

Faced with, or rather engulfed by, a work of this kind, one has to choose whether to follow the kaleidoscopic thematic traces suggested by the materials used (which relate to violence, pain, and trauma) or to let oneself go and experience it naively, using a kind of negative capability, or rather, as Nadia Fusini[9] writes, *another* capability. The point seems to be not so much to investigate ideology, religious fanaticism, and violence; nor does it deal in social criticism, good intentions, political activism, utopia, intellectual provocation, nationalism in India, and feminism. Instead, the important thing is to delve into the black heart of the self, into its aesthetic constitution, as it were at a pre-reflective stage, when it is still in the state of a magmatic and formless intersubjectivity.

Unsurprisingly, Nalini Malani's installation came to mind a few years later, in January 2015, at a Chris Ofili exhibition at the New Museum in New York entitled *Night and Day*. At some point, visitors to the show entered a large room bathed in half-light. They could barely make out the few large panels hanging on the walls. Adapting one's eyes to darkness was not enough to distinguish the images that were painted there. It was only by moving slowly that the outlines of large and disturbing figures could be made out through the slightest play of light produced by artfully arranged spotlights, and even then never in their entirety. In this way, the device invented by Ofili revealed the invisible and aroused feelings of awe and reverence. This happened not only because of the nature of the subjects painted but also because the spectator's extraordinary experience of interaction itself became the image of a vision so hopelessly solitary and precarious that it appeared to be part of a world of shadows.

Notes

1 N. Malani, *In Search of the Vanished Blood*, Documenta (13), Hatje Cantz Verlag, Ostfildern, 2012.

2 C. Wolf, *Cassandra*, 1984, transl. by J. van Heurck, Daunt Books, London, 2013.

3 R. M. Rilke, *The Notebooks of Malte Laurids Brigge*, 1910, transl. by M. Hulse, Penguin, London, 2009. See B.-C. Han, *Saving Beauty*, cited, p. 34: "In *The Notebooks of Malte Laurids Brigge*, Rilke describes seeing as an injury. Seeing exposes itself totally to what enters into the unknown zones of my ego. Thus, learning how to see is anything but an active, conscious process. Rather, it is a *letting-happen* or an *exposing-oneself-to-what-happens*".

4 H. Müller, "Die Hamletmaschine", 1977, transl. by C. Weber, *Performing Arts Journal*, Vol. 4, No. 3, 1980, pp. 141–146.

5 S. Beckett, *Krapp's Last Tape*, 53–63, 1958, in *The Collected Shorter Plays*. Grove Press, New York, 1984.

6 M. Devi, "Draupadi", 19–38, in *Breast Stories*, 1977, transl. by. C. Chakravorty Spivak, Seagull Books, Calcutta, 1997.https://archive.org/details/draupadi_202005/mode/2up

7 As outlined in Lévi-Strauss's discussion of it in *The Savage Mind*, the *bricoleur* is someone who develops their own creative process by re-using existing objects that are simply *available* for purposes other than those

originally intended. The key words in the semantic field of *bricolage* are empirical, contingency, aetiology, improvisation, play, occasion, shrewdness, flexibility, movement, adaptability, dilettantism (in the noble sense of cultivating an art not as a trade but for reasons of pleasure, passion, dedication and constancy). There is no need for "the equipment and knowledge of all trades and professions" (Devi, "Draupadi", p. 19). This does not mean that there is no logic or method in the process, but rather, as in the case of deconstruction, the method and logic involved are appropriate to the goal, at the same time as being extremely rigorous.

8 F. F. Coppola, *Apocalypse Now*, USA 1979.

9 See Fusini, N. (2016) "Another Capability, a Negative One". *The Italian Psychoanalytic Annual* 10:51–60. Taken from Keats, for W. R. Bion the concept of negative capability (and faith) becomes a principle of technique: the analyst must listen to the patient by abandoning memory, desire and understanding in order to heighten her receptivity to the productions of the unconscious. On this point, see G. Civitarese, "On Bion's concepts of negative capability and faith", *Psychoanalytic Quarterly*, 88, 751–783, 2019.

7

SAVAGE BEAUTY

When it comes to talking about Alexander McQueen, it is impossible to separate the life and tragic end of the designer from his work. Curated by Andrew Bolton and Harold Koda, the *Savage Beauty*[1] exhibition opened at the Metropolitan Museum in New York in February 2011. The year before, McQueen had committed suicide at the age of 40 in his Mayfair flat, just a week after the death of his mother Joyce, and on the eve of her funeral. In 2015, the exhibition then moved to London, to the Victoria and Albert Museum. Both of the exhibitions proved to be record-breaking events. There were hour-long queues to get in, the run of the exhibition was extended and it was even kept open throughout the night for the last two weekends. Incredible numbers of people who had never had an interest in fashion parades and who had previously not even known of McQueen's existence fell under the magnetism of a unique show.

Savage Beauty was the apotheosis of the career not just of a designer but of an artist. And, like all great artists, McQueen was the creator of a world at once ancient and totally new. His "landscapes" showed an ability to transfigure the most varied influences: Victorian London and skinhead London, the figure of his taxi driver father and the gay "underground" of Soho, his cockney roots and the working class, *Taxi Driver* and *The Shining*, Savile Row and the symbiotic bond with his mother, Elizabethan theatre and Yoruba mythology, *A Midsummer Night's Dream* and tattoos, the punk look and Givenchy; and then Damien Hirst, Matthew Barney and Leigh Bowery, but also the desperation that can be heard in the timbre of Michael Jackson's voice. All these elements – and many others – converge in McQueen's declared intention to use fashion to explore the dark side of personality, the invisible that hides beneath the visible, *the blood that courses under the skin*.

 DOI: 10.4324/9781003478904-7

Transgressive, provocative, obsessive, perfectionist, fragile, solitary, brilliant, *enfant terrible*, misogynist, depressed, "hooligan" – these are some of the adjectives that come to mind when thinking of McQueen. But why add him to the ranks of Serra, Kapoor, Malani, and Kiefer? Because like them he is someone who brilliantly transcended the boundaries of the field in which he worked. If we then consider that the order I have chosen to present these exemplars follows a gradient that ascends towards an ever more cogent explication of the psychological matrix that fashions this line of development, *Savage Beauty* shines out in all its disturbing luminosity.

While in *Torqued Ellipses* and *Symphony for a Beloved Sun* Kubin's spider-object remains enigmatic and the danger it represents is only hinted at, with McQueen the game being played gradually comes closer and closer to the surface. It is true that the same can of course be said of *In Search of Vanished Blood*. However, while Malani is interested in depths, for McQueen everything seems to lie on the surface. But that is only an illusion. What McQueen stages are not so much *cat walks* and are more akin to theatrical performances, but theatre *à la* Artaud, a theatre of cruelty; or, *à la* Grotowski, theatre as liturgy. His extraordinary ability lies not so much in creating clothes as in uncovering the fantasies present they conceal: the struggle for power, cruelty, the game played out between predator and prey, the sublime concurrence of ecstasy and agony, fear and pain.

In McQueen, the sublime weaves together romanticism and postmodernism, the monsters of 14th- and 15th-century Flemish painting, and the perverse world of serial killers in movies. The titles of some of his collections are statements of poetics. The first collection, with which he graduated from London's Central Saint Martins, was entitled *Jack the Ripper Stalks His Victims*, inspired by the serial killer who murdered five prostitutes in London in 1888. This choice served as a kind of template for all those to come. It was followed by *Taxi Driver, Nihilism, Highland Rape, Dante, Bellmer La Poupée*[2], *It's A Jungle Out There*; in 2010, *Angels & Demons*, and then, as in with Kapoor, numerous *Untitleds* (sometimes adopted to replace titles dropped because they considered too scandalous), right up to 2016 with *The Sea*. *The Birds*, on the other hand, was inspired by Hitchcock's memorable film of the same name, but also by Escher's drawings; *The Hunger* by a vampire film; *Elect Dissect* by H. G. Wells' novel *The Island of Dr. Moreau*, where the characters included animal-human hybrids. Other significant influences were Poe, Andreas Vesalius's anatomical drawings, Mary Shelley's *Frankestein*, Pasolini's *Salò, or the 120 Days of Sodom*, and Joel-Peter Witkin's photographs.

Larger than the show in New York, the London version of *Savage Beauty* was divided into six galleries. A sumptuous, labyrinthine landscape housed in the ideal venue of the Victoria and Albert Museum. McQueen had once said that the V&A was somewhere he would like to be locked up in at night. Many of those who visited *Savage Beauty* might well have said the same thing. A cruel, perverse, regal, ruthless, yet irresistibly seductive world. A magnificent, exotic, and sinister theatrical spectacle, with a cast of women who neither speak nor move, wonderfully inaccessible, powerful, irresistibly distant, painfully provocative, *amazing* but unapproachable women; women of the "look but don't touch" variety – essentially, a principle of the sublime. Bloodthirsty queens, priestesses of mystery cults, faceless and sometimes even headless, alien beings, masters of terror, and ladies of the night. Women prostitutes or hybrid figures – bird women, deer women, unicorn women, sphinx women, hawk women, eagle women. Feathered and caged, clad in shells or marine molluscs. This is the way McQueen brings nature into his creations: in the form of feathers, crustaceans, grasshoppers, locusts, fossils, bones, minerals, deer antlers, etc. Everywhere we find mythological animals, figures from a highly original textbook of fantastic zoology.

Then comes the "tear": if in the first room visitors are greeted by a reassuring megavideo of McQueen's fashion shows, already in the second they are introduced to a world where necrophilia reigns. More than the others, with the second double-height gallery called the *Cabinet of Curiosities*, which brings to mind both the luxury storefronts to be found in big cities, from Via Condotti to the fetish-like Hèrmes store in Ginza, and the shelves and display cases that in medical museums used to house anatomical preparations in formalin, it is like entering a mind with its various compartments. What is there to find here? Video clips of parades, animated objects, sounds, voices, images. We are not far from the taxonomies of Cesare Lombroso, from the oddities of Krafft-Ebing's[3] *Psychopathia Sexualis* and Freud's "perverse polymorphous child", from the "partial objects" that populate the inner world described by Melanie Klein. More and more from the outside to the inside: fetish objects, torsos, heads, mysterious hairstyles, women/mannequins with ribs and vertebrae exposed as weapons, accessories with the softness of prostheses that could have come from Cronenberg's[4] *Crash*. Each *item* in its own box/display cabinet: the macabre work of a perverse collector. The body is dissected, dismembered, and obsessively hunted through for a key to its understanding; to discover how to elude the insidiousness of the desperate desire aroused by beauty. Visitors to the exhibition are like so many Hiroshis, the medical student who is the main character in *Vital*, by Shinya Tsukamoto[5], and who finds himself dissecting the corpse of Ryôko, an ex-girlfriend who has died in a car accident, during an anatomy class. A game of perpetual metamorphoses. The same always comes back the same and always different. Self-evidently, however, the obsession with death is an obsession with life.

So *death*, then. Right from the very cover of the catalogue death is presented as the emblem of the exhibition: a hologram in which a skull is superimposed on the designer's face in an ambiguous interplay of the visible and the invisible, while the fashion show with the chess game is an obvious revisiting of Bergman's *The Seventh Seal*. In short, McQueen is unsurpassed in the way he brings together beauty and a sense of the macabre, for example, in the spectral hologram of Kate Moss dressed in white silk organza that closes the exhibition. It is not that there is no Grand-Guignol or kitsch in certain shock inventions, but, as Holland Cotter[6] notes in the *New York Times*, "everywhere there are arresting delicacies. The yellow-green beadwork is so fine it looks as soft as moss. Floral-patterned lace has been cut up, flower by flower, then stitched together again, but only partially, to give a dress the illusion of having being torn". Lastly, the parades of motionless mannequins cannot fail to call to mind the macabre dances to be found in so many Italian church frescoes.

Sometimes the fabric of the dress engulfs the whole head, "suffocating" it; sometimes the feet are mutilated; or then again a transversal cut between wrist and forearm or hip and belly catches the eye. Collars stretch upwards like sharp blades ready to cut. Some clothes would appear to be inspired by the Japanese erotic art of shibari. Other fabrics lend the mannequins a sense of movement that I feel I have only ever seen in the style of the dancers of the Lines Ballet in San Francisco, the ability to blend harmoniously with the whole through the astonishing fluidity of their movements. A Botticellian *primavera* transfigured into *drag queens* and *fetishized* Ophelias. Anatomical clothes, sutures of irredeemable scars; clothes-armour, clothes-ribs, clothes-shells for insect women.

Walking must be made difficult, impossible, painful (*sublime*). The fact is that shoes are not meant for walking, but for imparting a sublime thrust to the sacred, for insisting on an adoring[7], bottom-up vision. On these stilts, women levitate like unattainable goddesses. Not "walking", then, but deconstructing movement. Only in this way will their admirable architecture stand out and their sensuality and poignant beauty be enhanced.

The aim is to reveal the depth of surface. The patterns and colours of certain tight-fitting dresses could be mistaken for pages in an anatomical atlas. Sometimes a flap of clothing is lifted opening up a view of viscera because fabric and skin are one and the same. No longer tissue but parenchyma pleura, pericardium, mediastinum, ribs, kidneys, sternum, veins, arteries, and glands, peritoneum. In some places, the dummies in the catalogue show reddish streaks prompting one inevitably to think of blood; and where the senses fail to apprehend see it, it is the imagination that makes it visible; but only hidden by the tissue. As Barthes[8] observes, the most erotic part of a body is *"where the garment gapes"* the "skin glistening between two garments (the shirt and the trousers), between two edges (the half-open shirt, the glove and the sleeve); it is precisely this glitter that seduces, or even: the staging of an apparition-disappearance". But what unfolds here is an aesthetic and an *"eroticism of harm"*[9]: not the skin, or not just the skin, but what lies beneath: the radical passivity or "special sensitivity of the amorous subject, which makes him vulnerable, exposed to even the slightest wounds" of someone who, being "flayed [...] skinless, unprotected, resembling 'an undifferentiated ball of irritable substance' [...] the subject is totally painful and totally erotic [...] Sensitivity ends up existing as a form of being"[10].

In short, we gradually realize that the bodies dressed by McQueen are wounded and bleeding bodies. The actual title is *Savage Beauty*, but the title of Malani's installation, *In Search of Vanished Blood,* would work just as well. Even more than in the exhibition, the thematic element of blood is evident in the accompanying catalogue. As Judith Thurman[11] writes:

> The Norwegian fashion photographer Sølve Sundsbø took the catalogue pictures. It looks as though he bought the mannequins from a junk dealer, and it is startling to learn that they are live models disguised as dummies. Their bodies were coated with white acrylic makeup, and articulated at the joints by black strings. In the

retouching process, they lost their heads. But here and there—on a torso, a thigh, an arm—the makeup has worn away, and a bruise-like patch of pink skin shows through, as if the flesh of a corpse were coming to life. The freshness of the shock is pure McQueen.

One feature that is worth coming back to is the incredible attention McQueen paid to hair styles. McQueen even goes so far as to dress women in gowns made up of black hair gathered in swirls that descend over the whole body. There is nothing accidental about his "fetishistic" habit of signing his creations with a lock of hair enclosed in a translucent Perspex bag. The inspiration for this came to him from the custom that prostitutes in Victorian times had of selling their hair to make wigs. People who deal with children know that at a very young age, it is normal for them to stroke their mother's hair and to enjoy the special qualities it offers of being smooth, thin, strong, and soft. Sliding it slowly between thumb and forefinger, they seek its powerful hypnotic effect. Likewise they can take consolation and pleasure from a silk handkerchief or a simple piece of cloth. Winicott calls these "transitional" objects, located somewhere between the imaginary and the real. It is easy to conjecture that this sensitivity to the bodily matter of the object can become an acute sensitivity to scents, to the shininess and sumptuousness of fabrics, to sounds. As emerges clearly from Süskind's[12] and Schneider's[13] novels, a traumatic core often lies behind an artistic vocation. And yet hair by definition becomes one of those elements of the body (as is the case with nails, blood, semen, menstruation, vomit, saliva, pus, sweat, urine, etc.) that become abject as soon as they are separated from it.

After all, McQueen is a great hypochondriac. The hypochondriac suffers from sense, not meaning. The crisis of sense (that which imparts strength and direction to the subject) is always a crisis of affectivity. Hence the merciless scrutiny of the body: because suddenly the 'written' body becomes unreadable. The fact is that the body proper (sensible, legible, directed) arises from identification with the object. By "fetishizing" a particular organ, the hypochondriac rummages in around in his own flesh and what he finds is not his own body but that of the other. Similarly, a lover scrutinizes the beloved's face in order to decipher its expression. Like the lover-diagnostician, the hypochondriac is a visionary capable of hallucinoses, in other words, sensitive intuitions of states of affairs that cannot be grasped with the senses. At its most extreme, Roland Barthes[14] suggests, this scholarly gaze can "go from the *in vivo* to the *in vitro*, that is, make the other's body inert, and wish to possess this inertia. Not sadism, since the Sadian victims should cooperate and even rejoice, but rather necrophilic drive". Could one then say that necrophilic passion, as seen in certain films about serial killers, for instance in *The Cell*[15], is the malignant and hyperbolic stage of hypochondriac anxiety?

Notes

1 A. Bolton, ed., *Alexander McQueen: Savage Beauty,* Metropolitan Museum of Art, New York – Yale University Press, New Haven, CT 2011.

2 The same imagery fascinated Freud (Freud, S. (1919) "The 'Uncanny'". The Standard Edition of the Complete Psychological Works of Sigmund Freud 17:217–25) when he wrote about Hoffmann's short story, "The Sand Wizard", with its robot-women Olympia and Clara. See A. Moroni, *Sul perturbante. Attualità e trasformazioni di un'idea freudiana nella società e nella clinica psicoanalitica di oggi*, Mimesis, Milan-Udine 2019. See also Longinus, *On the Sublime*, cited, pp. 205–207: "One may indeed very well make an exception where the effect required is one of commiseration or depreciation, but in all other forms of amplification to remove the touch of sublimity is like taking soul from body. For their practical effect instantly loses its vigour and substance if it is not reinforced by the strength of the sublime"; and further, p. 217: "the object of the poetical form is to enthral [but ἔκπληξις also means "terror" or "consternation]".

3 R. von Krafft-Ebing, *Psychopathia Sexualis*, 1886, transl. by C. G. Chaddock, The F. A. Davis Company, Philadelphia, 1894, https://archive.org/details/PsychopathiaSexualis1000006945/page/n5/mode/2up?view=theater (accessed Dec. 5th, 2022).

4 D. Cronenberg, *Crash*, Canada and Great Britain 1996.

5 S. Tsukamoto, *Vital*, Japan 2004.

6 H. Cotter, "Designer as dramatist, and the tales he left behind", *The New York Times*, May 4, 2011: https://www.nytimes.com/2011/05/07/arts/design/alexander-mcqueen-show-at-the-met-review.html?pagewanted=all&_r=0 (accessed Sep. 16th, 2020).

7 H. Cotter, "Designer as dramatist, and the tales he left behind", cited, my italics: "Designer as dramatist, and the tales he left behind", cit.: "The platform boots that go with the suit are amazing. Curved like giant hooves, or like ballet slippers grotesquely frozen on point, they make an unforgettable sight, as sculpture should. *They're functionally cruel, formally perfect, conceptually wild.* If you can walk in them at all, and apparently some people can, they have to change the way you move through the world".

8 R. Barthes, *The Pleasure of the Text*, 1973, transl. by R. Miller, Hill and Wang, New York, 1998, p. 9.
9 Han, B.-C. Han, *Saving Beauty*, cited, p. 33.
10 R. Barthes, *Il discorso amoroso. Seminario a l'École Pratique des Hautes Études 1974–1776, seguito da Frammenti di un discorso amoroso (previously un published)*, 2007, It. tr. by A. Ponzio, Mimesis, Milan–Udine 2015, pp. 465–466.
11 J. Thurman, "Dressed to thrill: Alexander McQueen at the Met", *The New Yorker,* https://www.newyorker.com/magazine/2011/05/16/dressed-to-thrill (accessed Sep. 2th, 2019)
12 P. Süskind, *Perfume: The Story of a Murderer*, 1985, transl. by J. E. Woods, Vintage, New York, 2001.
13 P. Schneider, *Brother of Sleep*, 1992, transl. by S. Whiteside, The Overlook Press, New York, 1995.
14 R. Barthes, *Il discorso amoroso. Seminario a l'École Pratique des Hautes Études 1974–1776, seguito da Frammenti di un discorso amoroso (previously unpublished)*, cited, p. 472.
15 T. Singh, *The Cell*, cited. See also the chapter on this movie in G. Civitarese, 2013, *The Necessary Dream: New Theories and Techniques of Interpretation in Psychoanalysis*. Routledge, London, 2014.

8

HEAVENLY PALACES

Mounted in 2004 at the Hangar Bicocca, formerly a Pirelli factory, Anselm Kiefer's permanent installation *The Seven Heavenly Palaces 2004-2015* consists of seven concrete and lead towers varying in height from 13 to 19 metres, each weighing approximately 90 tonnes, and five large poly-material canvases. The various buildings are inspired by the 5th–6th century CE Jewish treatise Sefer Hekhalot (Book of Palaces). The names of the towers are: *Sefiroth*, *Melancholia*, *Ararat*, *Magnetic Field Lines*, *JH & WH*, and *Tower of Falling Pictures*. With the exception of Sefiroth, all towers are leaning and consist of five to a maximum of seven levels represented by modules made from containers used as formwork. Each module has some blind walls and some with openings. The side on which they open varies. In addition, there are sometimes traces of an original red or blue colour.

In an interview, Kiefer[1] explained that at some point he "started stacking 'L' shapes on top of each other like children do when they play with construction cubes". He talks about the fact that he was born during the war and that his childhood was one without toys: "the only things I could play with were the debris of our house, which had been bombed the night I came into the world. With those bricks I built houses, sometimes several storeys high, and inside I felt protected, whether it rained or the sun shone".

Painted between 2009 and 2013, the canvases were added later: *Jaipur*, two from the series *Cette obscure clarté qui tombe des étoiles*, *Alchemie*, and *Die deutsche Heilslinie*. The composition of this last painting is particularly interesting. The largest, albeit aesthetically the least successful, introduces a motif typical of the sublime: a solitary man with his back to the foreground gazes at an infinite landscape. The curve of a rainbow furrows the canvas across its full extent, connecting

DOI: 10.4324/9781003478904-8

heaven and earth. On its trajectory, one after the other, are listed the names of important German thinkers, from Kant to Marx, who expressed ideas on how to achieve a path to salvation for all mankind.

Each component part of the installation brings together numerous references. It would take a long time to list them all. Among the aspects that are of most interest to us in the context of our discussion about the contemporary sublime, the dimensions of the work are what stand out above all else. Like the works of Serra and Kapoor, *The Heavenly Palaces* are made to overpower, impress, intimidate, and fascinate. Again pride of place is occupied by the kinetic aspect. Here too, the viewer feels drawn to actively explore the space of the installation. He thus goes through a deeply immersive experience. The position of someone contemplating a painting, reading a book, listening to music or watching a film in the cinema is different, as these are all situations in which coenesthesia is more or less suspended.

Another key point: the theme of the divine is sublime in itself. Linked instead directly to the conceptual realm of psychoanalysis are the motifs of melancholy and creativity. The sense of danger emanating from the installation is present on several levels. Firstly, Ararat is a name linked to universal punishment, two towers (*JH & WH*) have to do with the prohibition against invoking the name of God (Jahweh), and melancholia brings to mind Freud's famous 1915 essay "Mourning and Melancholia". But more than that, the threat is an aesthetic experience. These buildings appear less than "heavenly" and they are in fact rather run-down. The structures give the impression of being really unsafe. The sense of intimidation is, as it were, real and by no means abstract.

The task of openly representing this aspect is carried out by the *Tower of Falling Pictures* to Stacked before the doorway at the bottom is a pile of wooden frames of various sizes covered in lead and containing crushed, dusty sheets of glass. One possible interpretation is that this accumulation of rubbish made up of common objects refers to the loss of emotional frames and conceptual categories. In this view, the particular detail would point to enacting the contemporary difficulty of reading the contexts of social reality due to the loss of traditional conceptual references. The fear, in short, would be that of losing the ability to represent, of feeling the divinity of language collapse in upon on us. Kiefer thus erects a majestic construction, but one that is on the verge of imploding in on upon itself[2]. After all, what else does it mean when we talk about the "death of God".

Inevitably, the theme of the confusion of tongues is intrinsic to the towers. But adducing multiple quotations is also a way of muddying the waters. Curiously, in 2010, the direction of the path through the exhibition was changed and now the panel with the map of the installation and the names of the buildings is at the end but closer to the exit. This makes it more difficult for those visiting the installation for the first time to make sense of it. When all is said and done the only tower that remains is the tower of the confusion of languages and the Babel of interpretations. The apocalyptic theme is therefore also central to the *Heavenly Palaces*[3]. It is catastrophe understood in the dual senses of destruction and regeneration. Moreover, this is what art always represents. Sometimes the one, sometimes the other.

The verticality and the theme of the divine clearly evoke the above-mentioned state of the infant's dependence on the adult, which is then extended to describe the dependence of the faithful on God[4]. As in Gothic cathedrals, ascent stands for the mystical journey. It is the dynamic summed up in the concept of *at-one-ment*: the act of atonement and reconciliation with God. Atonement for what? Evidently for something that has to do with hubris, excess, ὕβρις. This immediately brings us back to one of the typical archetypal motifs of the aesthetics of the sublime: ruins. What is it about ruins that we find so fascinating and frightening? Obviously not ruins per se, but the invisible presence of an immense power of destruction. The power to annihilate that we unconsciously cannot help but personify in the object on which we depend and which we always aspire to attain.

Melancholia, at the foot of the east side, displays thousands of small strips of glass and paper with handwritten alphanumeric sequences. They bring to mind Menashe Kadishman's *Shalecht* installation ("like fallen leaves") at the Jewish Museum in Berlin, one of the most powerful memorials to the Holocaust, in which visitors walk on ten thousand metal plates that look like faces deformed in a scream of pain. Similarly, it is difficult not to associate the ruinous appearance of the towers with the image of the only tower that survived the bombing of the Kaiser-Wilhelm-Gedächtniskirche in 1943, a church deliberately left in mutilated form as a symbol of the disasters brought about by arrogance[5], but also of the rebirth of the city. One is also reminded of the shantytown of containers stacked one on top of the other through which the U-Bahn sped in the 1990s on the gigantic construction site set up to rebuild Postdamer Platz under the direction of Renzo Piano.

The Seven Heavenly Palaces thus present various facets: the path of humility to mystical asceticism created through poor materials; obscurity as an initiatory path; the vertical self-representation beloved of those in power, especially when it tends to sacralize itself; presence imbued with absence and vice versa; the opposition between the visible and invisible, the external and the internal, the high and the low; catastrophe or the "threat of chaos"[6] but, at the same time, "resistance to chaos"[7]: in essence, all dimensions of the work necessary for the repair of the object that has been attacked in the unconscious fantasy.

Notes

1 "Anselm Kiefer in conversation with Giovanna Amadasi", in G. Amadasi, ed., *Anselm Kiefer's Seven Heavenly Palaces*, 55–59, Mousse Publishing, Milan 2018, p. 57.
https://pirellihangarbicocca.org/en/bubble/catalogue-extract-anselm-kiefer-in-conversation-with-giovanna-amadasi/ (accessed Dec. 6th, 2022)

2 See F. Vercellone, *Simboli della fine*, Il Mulino, Bologna 2019.

3 On the receptive-divinatory significance of the paradigm of the apocalypse, see S. Vitale, *La dimora della lontananza. Saggi sull'esperienza dello spazio intermedio*, Clinamen, Florence 2005.

4 See S. Freud, *The Future of an Illusion*, cited.

5 On the subject of arrogance, see the short yet scintillating paper by W. R. Bion, On Arrogance. *International Journal of Psychoanalysis* 39:144–146, 1958. The central idea is that arrogance springs from lack of recognition and the fear it produces.

6 D. W. Winnicott, "Mirror Role of Mother and Family in Child Development", 1971, pp. 149–159, in: *Playing and Reality*, Routledge, London, 2009, p. 171.

7 G. Guercio, "Numinosità e occultamento", pp. 19–51, in G. Amadasi (ed.) *Anselm Kiefer. I Sette Palazzi Celesti*, cit., p. 32.

9

CAN'T HELP MYSELF

> Out, damned spot! out, I say! [...]
> Yet who would have thought the old man to have had so much blood in him?
>
> Shakespeare, *Macbeth*

Visitors entering the central pavilion of the 58th edition of the Venice Biennale (2019) curated by Ralph Rugoff and entitled *May You Live in Interesting Times* found themselves immediately face to face with the fascinating and terrible spectacle[1] of an installation bearing the title *Can't Help Myself* (2016). Exhibited for the first time at the Guggenheim in New York on the occasion of the exhibition *Tales of our Time*, it was the work of Sun Yuan and Peng Yu, two "post-conceptual" artists already renowned for other provocative and unconventional works.

Inside a huge transparent acrylic cube, a kind of robot-monster moves rhythmically engaged in some mysterious compulsive activity. This strange technological being has grafted a mechanical arm similar to those used on car assembly lines or which form part of bulldozers onto a "body" that serves as its base. It swings it through the air with great agility, then places it on the ground and uses it to wipe away a copious, viscous, blood-dark liquid.

The machine is equipped with sensors for visual recognition and intervenes when it registers that the "blood" has flowed back beyond the boundaries of a predetermined area. The movement of this broad fishtail is centripetal in direction, but each time the plane is tilted, the liquid flows back in the opposite direction and away from the machine. In this way, a kind of perpetual wave motion is generated.

 DOI: 10.4324/9781003478904-9

With the container protecting the spectators, like a tiger's cage at the zoo, they become the true protagonists of the installation. What would be the point of erecting such barriers if not to include them as the main actors? It is from this It is as if they were hypnotized by the scene and thus recruited to become unwitting participants in a performance. By means of this necessary addition, a picture is composed in which we can find all the basic elements of the aesthetics of the sublime that we mentioned earlier.

The robot's supple, rhythmic movements – as many as 32 types are planned – are guided by a computer system. It is as if it were performing an absurd and fiercely ironic ballet. It does much more than perform movements designed to contain the liquid in a delimited space. Rather, at times it interrupts this repetitive and impossible task of creating order, its arm stretching upwards until it is completely extended. It is then as if it were making a gesture of triumph or perhaps protest or despair, or, perhaps even, chanting a kind of hymn. At such moments one might almost say that the strange monster-animal has something human about it. The actual squeals it emits do not seem to be coming from a pile of metal and electric wires.

The robot impresses with its strength, agility, endurance, and perseverance. As occurs in the most heinous murders, blood stains cover the walls. One is bound to ask: the traces of whose crime does the machine obsessively insist on washing away? Whose blood has been spilled? Whose labyrinth is the bloodthirsty guardian protecting? Who is the Lady Macbeth desperately trying to scrub her bloodstained hands clean?

The machine provides no answers and may arouse not only fear but also a certain pleasure. If we think of how many works in the same exhibition express themselves through the accumulation of materials, references, and quotations, what is striking here is how the artists achieve impressive effects with an extreme economy of means. This process of schematization, as of a life and a body summed up in a single gesture, is highly effective because it touches upon something primordial.

We have made the point that the machine seems to perform a ballet. But a "ballet" reminiscent of the installation was indeed staged recently at the Royal Opera House in London. I am referring to the dance-theatre performance created by Arthur Pita in 2011, *The Metamorphosis* (Fig. 9.1), obviously inspired by Kafka's famous novella, and now staged with a score by Frank Moon.

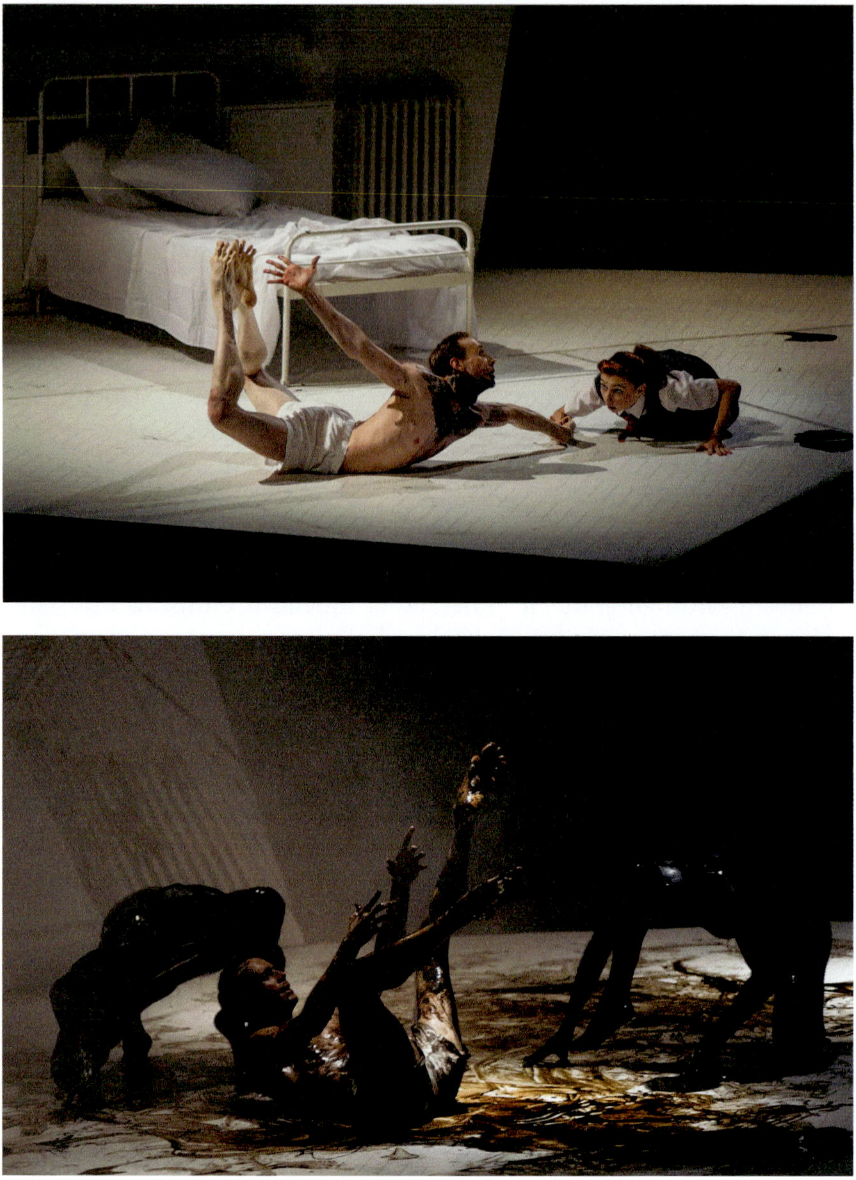

Fig. 9.1 A. Pita, *The Metamorphosis*, 2013 edition, Joyce Theater, New York

Edward Watson is exceptional in the part of Gregor Samsa. He brings off painstaking and astonishing contortions as he discovers his new identity as a repulsive insect. His mouth emits a dark viscous liquid that spreads across the floor and sticks to his whole body. The impression is that it is blood and that what we are witnessing is his slow bleeding to death. The stage space is arranged around the split between Gregor's room and the kitchen where his family members gather to witness his drama utterly at a loss to understand what is going on. This mirrors the separation-laceration that in *Can't Help Myself* correlates to the walls of the transparent box that isolates the machine from the spectators. If Kafka's story transports us from wakefulness into the hallucinated world of dreams and madness, the perturbing metamorphosis dreamt up by Yuan and Yu delves even deeper and presents itself as the hallucination of a hallucination.

Note

1 Anyone wishing to admire the "robot" in action can watch it online at https://www.youtube.com/watch?v=VPZ7lhNszvg

10

SUBLIMATION REINVENTED

Let us now try to sum up what we have been saying so far. We have seen that one of the characteristics of the sublime is the terror aroused by the object depicted in the works. While in McQueen, Malani, Yuan, and Yu, this feeling is clearly expressed, in Kapoor, Serra, and Kiefer, on the other hand, it is an enigmatic presence: for instance, it comes out in the risk of falling into the void, losing one's way in a labyrinth or being crushed by collapsing towers. The fact is that the object is also *terribly* attractive. If this were not the case, there would, as it were, be no story to tell. The subject would turn away hastily and that would be sufficient and as far as necessary. The point that the sublime embodies, however, is the situation in which the subject is unable to get too close, but neither can it move away, because it is firmly tied in with the object. Although the reason for wanting to move away from a ravine or an active volcano may be self-evident, it is more difficult to identify what constitutes the true nature of the object's fascination. This is the question that Kant, for example, attempts to answer. And he is only able to do so, intellectually, by situating it in the infinite quality characteristic of the depicted object and in the narcissistic gratification of the spectator who feels "superior"[1] by virtue of his ability to exercise rational dominion over it. But it is an answer that fails to satisfy and distracts us from something "obvious".

Indeed, the aesthetics of the sublime openly asserts that the reason it is impossible to keep one's distance lies in the unattainable beauty of the spectacle. Our task then is to equate this beauty more closely with a psychological necessity. What effect does beauty have on the way the mind is constructed? Why is feeding on it so vital to us? Why would it be just as dangerous not to do so as to let oneself

 DOI: 10.4324/9781003478904-10

be engulfed by waves or swept away by an avalanche? If we want to understand why moving away or getting closer would be two equally catastrophic outcomes that both involve losing oneself and the other, we must realize that beauty is *necessary* to life. Beauty, that which we experience as such, and therefore most notably beauty that comes to be sublime, encapsulates in itself the infinite series of events that in the relationship with the other are produced at the "molecular" level, and for this reason, it is synonymous with thought or the capacity to represent or depict.

My hypothesis is that the sublime is nothing other than the infinitely enlarged narrative derivative of a relational and dynamic emotional configuration that, as in a fractal, repeats itself gradually on an ascending scale of size. In my opinion, the only possible explanation why the spectator cannot move too far away from the represented object is because the pole of attraction lies not in the theme (the *what*) of the representation but in its form (the *how*). The aesthetic experience in art, which is then what is prompted by that form, is in all respects equatable with the aesthetic experience of unison (*at-one-ment*)[2] within the primary relationship – and then also in all other future relationships – that creates the mind [*fa mente*]. It is a moment of truth that makes the self-grow. How could one ever do without it?

Thus, the aesthetic pleasure enjoyed in the overall experience of giving in to the allure of a work of art, unconsciously only represents a balanced solution for the emotional dystonia caused by the fear of the object's absence (absence is not only abandonment but also "disappearance" through indifferentiation) and the irresistible fascination it exerts. After all, *fascinum* means both passion and malice, enchantment and evil spell. In other words, on the one hand, it represents the state of dependence, both material and moral, in which the child finds itself in relation to the object, since it depends on its care and is tied to it by a bond of love; on the other hand, in order to become a subject in its own right, it must detach itself from it.

In essence, it is the same position as that occupied by Professor Rath in relation to Lola Lola in Josef von Sternberg's[3] *The Blue Angel*, Mathieu with *Conchita* in Luis Buñuel's[4] *That Obscure Object of Desire*, the little boy contemplating the gigantic fading image of his mother's face in Ingmar Bergman's[5] *Persona* (Fig. 10.1), and Louise Banks facing the aliens[6] whose language she has been tasked to decipher in *Arrival*.

Of course, this does not enable us to give a more thorough account of how the mechanism of constructing the psyche works,

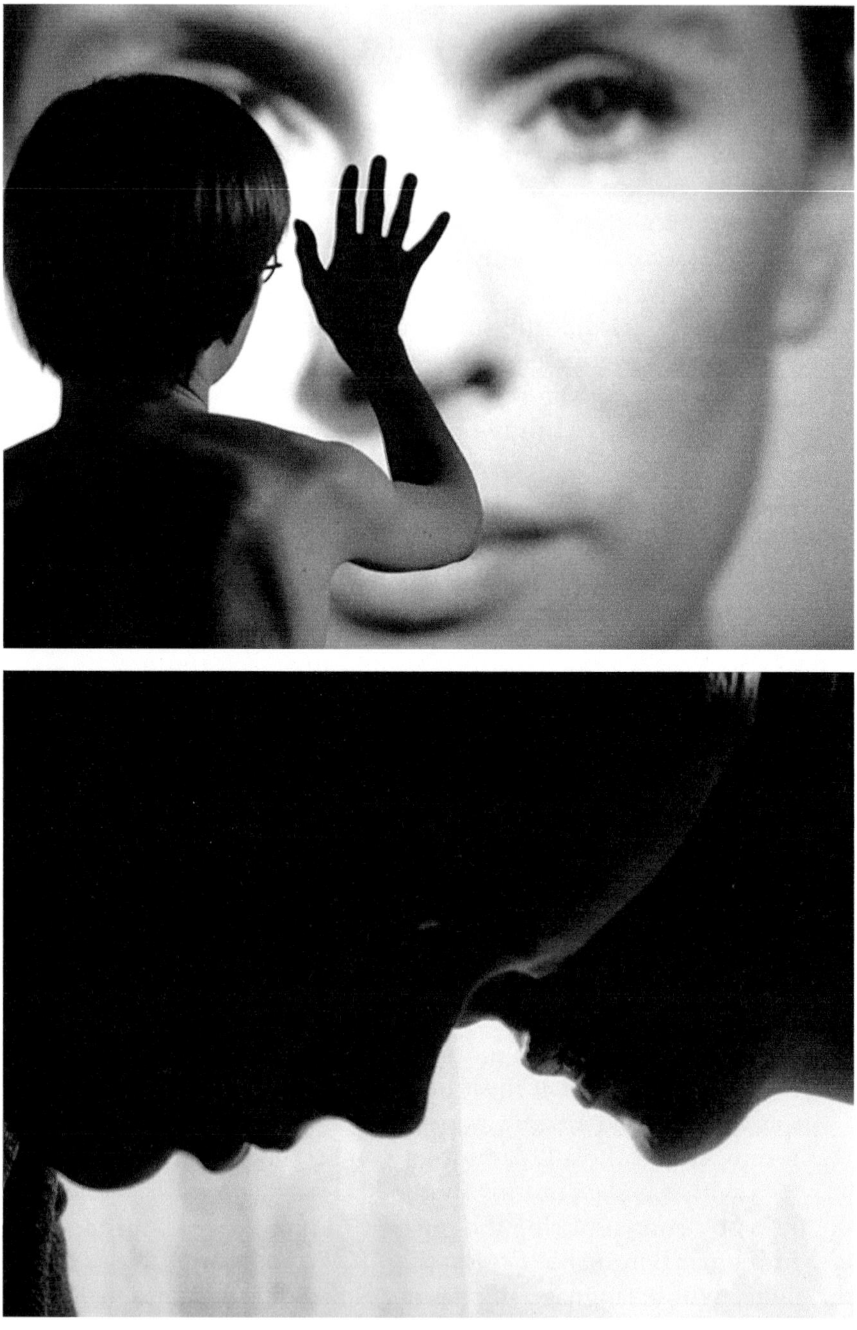

Fig. 10.1 I. Bergman, *Persona*, Sweden 1966

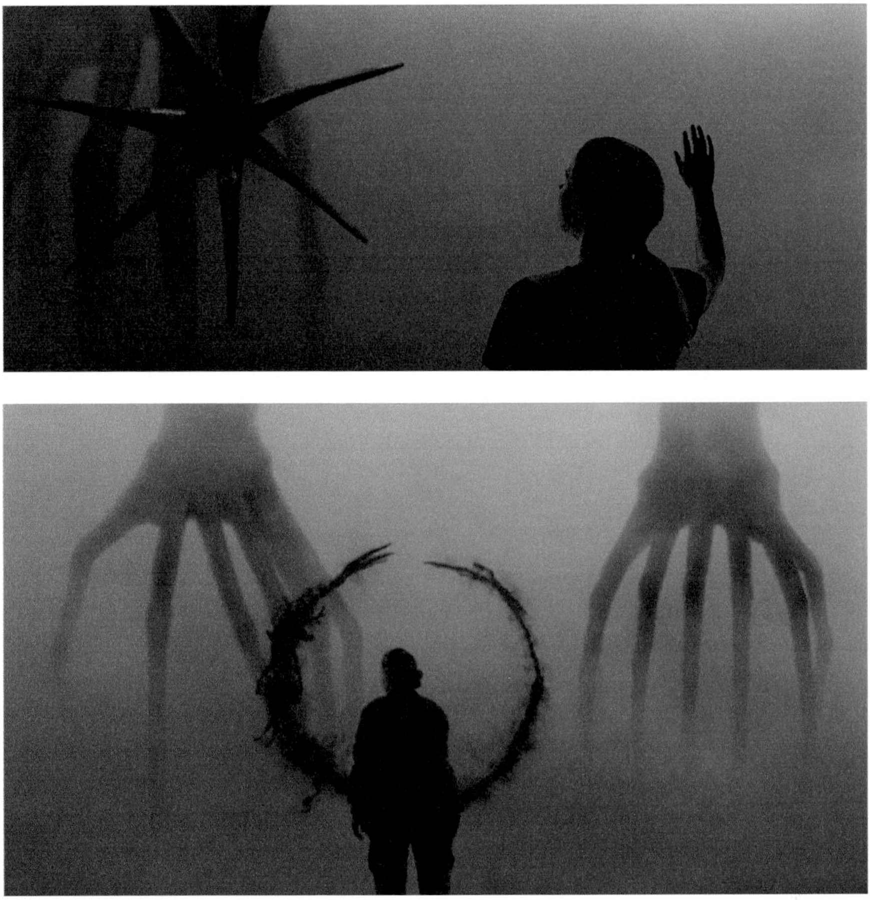

Fig. 10.2 D. Villeneuve, *Arrival*, USA 2016

which entails moments of attunement with the other, precisely because it involves layers of our being that are not thematic but sensory, affective, semiotic, and corporeal. Nor would it make sense to ask why we experience certain forms as beautiful. We would end up regressing to an infinity in which tautologically we could not assert anything beyond the notion that evidently it must be something instinctive, having to do with a certain order felt as revitalizing in the very materiality of "flesh", and so on.

We can seek to define the ultimate reasons that make what we experience beautiful and true, but essentially, we cannot "say" them. On these grounds, no aesthetic canon could ever satisfy us, despite all the attempts that have been made to settle on a definitive version. That said, psychoanalysis does help us penetrate a little into this secret by virtue of the courage (and often the "indispensable" recklessness) of its hermeneutic competence. This competence, which should not be overlooked, is coupled with a passion for empiricism. It is the famous Freudian *Junktim*[7]. The analyst always works in an experimental situation because potentially he listens to the patient's account of his own psychic suffering without setting any limits.

To further clarify some of the aspects we have already caught glimpses of, namely, the relationship in the sublime that the subject entertains with a superior or divine entity, and what the resulting feeling of moral uplift entails, or rather, how the repulsive movement of estrangement prompted by the feeling of danger is associated with a movement of "ascent". The first psychoanalytic concept that comes to mind is sublimation. To my knowledge, no one has ever seriously related the aesthetic concept of the sublime to the psychoanalytic concept of sublimation. This could be because the former is still relevant today, while the latter, although it has entered common parlance, has become somewhat marginal. Yet both contain the idea of a device, rhetorical and psychic, respectively, that takes the subject to new heights in the process of his own self-fulfillment. The intersection of two seemingly heterogeneous terms helps us to fruitfully encroach on disciplinary boundaries and to reread the vicissitudes of the primary relationship by "pretending" that sublime literature or sublime painting are cryptic yet highly effective illustrations of it.

Coined by Freud in 1897 in the context of the case of *Dora*, the term sublimation serves to indicate a kind of hydraulics of drive energy. Instead of discharging itself directly into sexual satisfaction, this "fluid" is channelled towards other goals that society regards as of considerable value. The new goal is psychically akin to the old but "higher and consequently unobjectionable"[8]. It has greater social value because it specifically concerns human and socially approved functions and activities. Sublimation is thus a "transformed passion", in which the force of the drive has been mitigated, "tamed"[9] and its direction diverted. It aims at a "finer and higher" joy, albeit of much lower intensity than the direct satisfaction of the cruder drives, and such that "it does not shake our bodily existence". As a concept, sublimation is therefore a kind of two-faced Janus. On the one hand, it clarifies the dynamics of a particular defence (one exchanges the no longer legal currency of sexual gratification for recognition); on the other hand, it serves as a model of how man can accomplish the scientific, artistic, and cultural achievements for which he is most admired and of which he is most proud.

In the concept of sublimation, Freud merely sums up the central thesis of *Civilization and its Discontents*: every superior and shared spiritual achievement stems from partially forgoing the satisfaction of instinctual needs; civilization is based on repression. The formula is intuitive and illuminating; however, if we look inside ourselves with a spirit untainted by preconceptions, we begin to ask questions. For instance, when he postulates the absolute freedom of the animal world, Freud appears to be establishing a myth. What freedom can one ever speak of with regard to animality? It would be like imagining that there are no constraints, such as do in fact exist, which are far more rigid, even if they are not cultural but merely biological. The idea of a totally free Eden and the acquisition of language and self-consciousness as a fall is nothing other than our own projection. In this Eden, of course, we imagine ourselves restored to the original completely guilt-free condition of pure and free beings, just as we think animals are free to enjoy everything without constraint[10]. But animals are by no means free; as Heidegger says, they are "poor in world". And if, then, man gains more freedom, it is hard to see why this should not also apply to the sphere of sexuality in general. Could it not then be said that having transformed instinct into drive has not repressed but liberated sexuality that is no longer animal? Are we really sure that happiness is the price to be paid for civilization?

But the problems with sublimation do not stop here. It is not clear how the drive can change from being sexual to being non-sexual, where the dividing line lies between sublimation, normality, and pathology; nor is the line clear between minimal, "everyday" sublimation and the actual ability to bring an artistic creation to life. If, as Freud says, it is a solution "accessible only to a few", does this greatly limit its explanatory power; or is it then something that concerns everyone?

The concept of sublimation in Freud thus identifies "one of the lacunae in psycho-analytic thought"[11]. It is a problematic concept. If we want to deploy it to understand the sublime, we have to reinvent it. How can we do this? By taking an alternative route. We can take "sublimation" to mean the act of rising above animality that can only be based on inter-human agreement and the creation of the intermediate space of language[12]. This would make it synonymous with "abstraction", i.e. the process whereby we obtain abstract concepts or ideas. The concepts of language allow us to rise above animality (or put distance between ourselves and the object, which, from another point of view, is the same thing).

The signs in our living environment enable us to categorize it, and thus simplify experience by discovering analogies between different terms, and to access new cognitive levels. We gain self-awareness. In itself, language works on the one hand by giving us the opportunity to experience ourselves as finite and individuated because it offers us the fiction of having an *I* and a *now*, but on the other hand, it exposes us to the perturbing effect of being infinite because we are "spoken" by the ever-expanding infinity of language. It would not be wrong to say that the grandeur that Kant emphasizes in the aesthetics of the sublime and that is allegorized by the landscape of nature is the system of language as infinite. The *I/group* dialectic is thus found in the finite/infinite dialectic. As Martin Buber[13] writes,

> The responsibility of every man is an infinite sphere, it is responsibility before the infinite. Man moves, he speaks, he looks, and each of his movements, each of his words, each of his glances moves the happening of the world, without him knowing how strong and wide are the waves of that motion. With all his being and acting, each man determines the fate of the world to an extent unknowable to him, because the causality we can perceive is but a tiny segment of the invisible action, unimaginable in its multiplicity, that everyone exerts upon everyone. Thus *every human act is a vessel of infinite responsibility*.

Addressing the relationship between the finite (where the subject assumes responsibility for the act he performs) and the infinite (which means the impossibility of consciously assuming *all* responsibility for it) is tantamount to questioning the birth of the psyche, a subject on which contemporary – now post-Freudian – psychoanalysis has been working hard, and with interesting results. But then we immediately come up against obstacles: if the child cannot speak, what process of "abstraction" is possibly involved? Intersubjective agreement (emotional attunement, moment of encounter, unison, *at-one-ment*, etc., all events that we can think of as moments of recognition, as finding an analogy, a factor of similarity between different individuals) cannot only be about pure spirit, abstract rationality; it must also – and originally must necessarily be – above all else "aesthetic" (affective, somato-psychic). In the beginnings of life (the Rilkean "principle of the terrible"), it concerns the thinking of the body (patterns, habits, bodily intentionality). Sublimation as a theory of subjectivation and the aesthetics of the sublime in art come together at this point. The trait shared by the two concepts is the emphasis on the foundational role of aesthetic intersubjectivity for human subjectivity. The thing to do, then, in order to return to the subject of sublimation is to rediscover the substantial and deep-seated equivalence between the aesthetic sublime and the psychological sublime. We need to emphasize the role of *form*, the single factor that, still central in Longinus, then begins to fade in authors who accentuate the psychological significance of the sublime and differentiate it from the beautiful.

The ascent to self-awareness that the (reinvented) concept of sublimation illustrates helps us to recognize in the art of the sublime the figurative account of the primary relationship with the object. The theoretical benefit is reciprocal. In the typical scene that the sublime recounts every time, the concept of sublimation helps us understand the process of the intersubjective constitution of the psychic. Weaving together the sublime and sublimation then brings other advantages. In return, what the allegory of the primary relation emphasizes in sublimation, centred as it is on the aesthetics of the encounter, is this "aesthetic" dimension as the substance of a new concept of sublimation.

The juxtaposition of the sublime and sublimation is far from being spurious. Enshrined within the words, what they have in common is the fact that they not only have the ascending trajectory that rises from the body to a morally higher vision but also the specific reference to art. Sublimation theory *is* the Freudian theory of the meaning of art. In the psychoanalytic literature on sublimation, clinical vignettes almost always show patients "sublimating" their repressed impulses into some more or less successful artistic activity. If, on the other hand, we look at the sublime in art, we do not find the connection to the need for consensual validation expressed so clearly. Certainly, a work of art is undoubtedly a social fact; the very definition of what in a given period is to be considered art or not art obeys precise cultural rules which are open to change. But only psychoanalytic reflection is able to bring into cogent focus the fact that the aesthetic experience represents a moment of communion with the other, a moment of relational construction of the self.

The circle, so to speak, closes. Sublimation, which in any case is explicitly tied in with the primary relationship with the object, with its vicissitudes and with its reissues and reprints, seems to us to be exemplarily narrated in the *topoi* of art inspired by the sublime; conversely, the *aesthetics* of the sublime helps us to theorize the (in the strictest sense of the word, aesthetic) plane of sensations on which the first ignition of subjectivity occurs. The hermeneutic step that needs to be taken to interweave the two concepts is obviously to read them, as it were, against the light and so as to perceive in the content and form of the work of art the design of the subject-object structure of the primary relationship and the dynamics that characterize it. This can be expressed by drawing on the recurrent subjects of painting inspired by the sublime: not (only) lava but contact with an object that burns; not (only) the glacier but the chilling gaze of a mother who does not instil vitality; not (only) monumental ruins but the abyss of abandonment, and so on. In certain cases, the interpretation is suggested by the subject of the painting itself.

It is the point we could sum up in the headword "anatomy", the last in our provisional lexicon of the sublime, and which actually stands for the transition from the objective body (*Körper*) to the lived body (*Leib*) or "affective body". For example, certain wild, hypnotic gorges resembling vaginas, as in Karl Friedrich Schinkel's 1818 *Felsentor* [*Rock Arch*], or, from the same year, the aforementioned *The Bridge of Varallo*, by Marco Gozzi, or, as we have seen, Turner's *The Parting of Hero and Leander*. Nature that becomes human when suffused with emotion allegorizes the transition from behaviour based on the automatic instinctuality of animals to behaviour based on self-awareness and reflection. But let us delve a little further into the psychoanalytic myth of psychic birth and the interweaving of the finite and the infinite that comes about through the word.

Notes

1 See B.-C. Han, 2015, *Saving Beauty*, cited, p. 21.

2 E. Munafò, *Il sublime e il modernismo. Eliot, Joyce, Woolf*, Carocci, Rome 2017, finds a similar concept in James Joyce's "epiphanies", Virginia Woolf's "moments of being", and T. S. Eliot's "timeless moments". Such moments of encounter or *at-one-ment* are both "sublime" if we look at the quotient of "affection" that constitutes their matter, and "sublimated" in the sense of the chemical metaphor of products of intersubjective refinement/simplification that ascends to level of the divine

of the concept. Affect is to be understood as an inherently intersubjective phenomenon. On this, see also M. Croce, *Postcritica. Asignificanza, materia, affetti*, Quodlibet, Macerata, 2019, pp. 74–75: "it is never the affair of a single body [...] but expresses the production of a new body from two or more bodies".

3 J. V. Sternberg, *The Blue Angel*, Germany, 1930.

4 L. Buñuel, *That Obscure Object of Desire*, Spain and France, 1987.

5 I. Bergman, *Persona*, Sweden, 1966.

6 D. Villeneuve, *The Arrival*, USA, 2016.

7 Cf. S. Freud, "The Question of Lay Analysis". The Standard Edition of the Complete Psychological Works of Sigmund Freud 20:177–258, 1926, p. 256: "In psycho-analysis there has existed from the very first an inseparable bond between cure and research. Knowledge brought therapeutic success. It was impossible to treat a patient without learning something new; it was impossible to gain fresh insight without perceiving its beneficent results. Our analytic procedure is the only one in which this precious conjunction is assured. It is only by carrying on our analytic pastoral work that we can deepen our dawning comprehension of the human mind. This prospect of scientific gain has been the proudest and happiest feature of analytic work".

8 S. Freud, *Five Lectures on Psycho-analysis*. The Standard Edition of the Complete Psychological Works of Sigmund Freud 11:1–56, 1910, p. 28.

9 S. Freud, *Civilization and its Discontents*, cited, p. 79.

10 On this point, see M. Bonazzi & D. Tonazzo, *Lacan e l'estetica. Lemmi*, Mimesis, Milan-Udine, 2005.

11 J. Laplanche & J.-B. *The Language of Psychoanalysis*, cited, p. 433.

12 See G. W. F. Hegel, *Phenomenology of Spirit, cited,* cit., pp. 308–309: "Language, however, contains it in its purity, it alone expresses the 'I', the I' itself. This *real* existence of the 'I' is, *qua* real existence, an objectivity which has in it the true nature of the 'I'. The 'I', is this particular 'I'—but equally the *universal* 'I'; its manifesting is also at once the externalization and vanishing of *this* particular 'I', and as a result the 'I' remains in its universality. That it is *perceived* or *heard* means that its *real existence dies away;* this its".

13 M. Buber, *Storie e leggende chassidiche*, It. tr. by A. Lavagetto, G. Bemporad, E. Broseghini, Mondadori, Milan 2008, p. 419, my italics.

11

THE MATTER OF TIME

The myth that psychoanalysis recounts obsessively is about how thought is born from the primary relation with the object; how the matter of time is generated. What counts more than anything else in this inaugural act whereby the mind is born from another mind and their "experience of being loved [*Liebeserfahrung*]"[1] is that an original temporality is founded on the regular interplay between the absence and presence of the object. It is clear that in order for this to work and for the rhythmic pattern of displeasure/pleasure to be established (or rather displeasure/non-displeasure), the main thing is not the search for pleasure but keeping pain away. The encounter both with the *other* as a concrete individual and care-giver, and with the *Other* as the unconscious, language, sociality, and culture is an absolutely essential precondition.

Thought, as Bion explains, arises out of the capacity to tolerate frustration: both the frustration caused by the absence that in itself dialectically contains the trace of presence, and by the absence that is contained as a trace in any presence. The symbol thus comes into being as a result of doing without the full presence of the object; in return, it proposes itself as a versatile tool for modulating the frustration that arises from doing so. "The hour of the sublime", to take up the title of an essay by Barnett Newman[2] *The sublime is now*, from the point of view of psychoanalysis is the "now" of the feeling of time, thus the hour of birth. If we deconstruct this "now", we see that it is made up of an original temporality that can, as it were, be read between the lines in terms of its intersubjective constitution. Now is first and foremost an abstraction, something we can *name*. If we did not have the word for "now", we could neither put a name on it or even "apprehend" it.

DOI: 10.4324/9781003478904-11

In the examples of the contemporary sublime that we have been examining so far, the extraordinary immersiveness of the aesthetic experience is exactly the same as that of *now*. These works are the equivalent of the virtual reality environments that are now deployed as concrete aids in various fields, for example, in museums and or in archaeology. What is essential is the naturalness of the medium of interaction. In "embodiments", buttons and keyboards disappear and become one with the body[3]. The fact that there is no visible interface lends a sense of naturalness and vividness to the experience, as happens when we move in the space-time containers of our everyday lives. But if, from a psychological point of view, we trace the feeling of the now back to the experience of being contained by the object, that is to say, when we manage to make sense of things, what we continue to experience is nothing other than the activity of precisely this internalized function which is now in the form of self-containment. On the level of fantasy, we are constantly immersed in the archaic world of the primary relation. From this point of view, aesthetic experience is a way of papering over the cracks in this essential and foundational structure of being; the aesthetic function of immersiveness is the unconscious simulacrum of a condition of fusion with the maternal body; finally, the very element of *pàthos* – both in the contents of the sublime and in the passion of the language necessary to express them – is a reflection of the "passionate" atmosphere that the infant breathes at birth in contact with the object.

Logically, the conclusion we have come to is that what is represented in aesthetic experience in general, in the experience of both the merely beautiful and the sublime, seen therefore as different gradations of the same phenomenon, is nothing other than the trauma of our own birth. The now, as a noun, connects the two non-existents of past and future, in the same way that the sign connects the two non-existents, if taken in isolation, of signifier and signified. We find here our moment of vertigo now identified with being, i.e. nothingness. The noun, which if it is to have meaning in its value as a linguistic sign can only represent the dimension of alienation that dwells in the subject, is the needle that constantly weaves the thread of past and future memories. As each new intersubjective knot is tied, more subjectivity is created. Each time the noun releases the subject from its entrapment in the *claustrum* of the maternal body and returns it to sociality. This is the true meaning I would now attribute to the Freudian concept of sublimation.

Standing in contrast to immersiveness is interaction. By this term we can mean everything that alerts us to the pretense of frames, contexts, *parergon*[4], and in the ultimate analysis to the fabric of the ego, to the risk of becoming too immersed in the relationship and thus losing ourselves. Interaction guards us against the danger of merging with the object and has an individuating function; or rather, individuation arises from the interplay of immersion and interaction, of presence and absence. More precisely, time as the possibility of living and saying "now" is both a psychic and a "somatic" concept, and thus, like any intersubjectively mediated concept of the melody of gratification and frustration, that is, of the object's presence and absence (or, rather, of the object's partially absent presence and partially present absence). Not only an ideational abstraction, therefore, but also a sensorial or corporeal abstraction, although without language this would be a necessary but not sufficient condition.

In essence, this is the question that the aesthetics of the sublime delves into in such an exemplary manner. It reveals and "theorizes" that the process of subjectivation understood as the progressive elevation of the individual from the chaos of unorganized instinctual experience to the socially ordered ("divine") plane of the concept and language not only takes place on a purely "signifying" or cognitive plane, but also on a sensory, affective, bodily, unsaturated, opaque level. The concept exists not only in an abstract, notional, or representative sphere but also in a sphere that is a practical, affective, bonding and operational.

Beauty of form thus corresponds to the perfect balance of thought. Thinking implies a certain pleasure. To be more precise: the pleasure of those who obscurely realize that beneath them lies the abyss of the loss of meaning, but in the meantime grab hold of the railing provided by the play of signifiers. For Barthes[5], "the writer is someone who plays with his mother's body", and for Pontalis[6], the dreamer reunites with his mother's body. But even before the act of "writing", "thinking" already holds a similar significance. If acquiring an original temporality, and then by turn the possibility of thinking, has to do with the child's primary relationship with the breast (notably with the establishment of an orderly rhythm of gratification and frustration that is then "filmed" in a noun), then thinking is really like playing blind man's buff with the mother's body – with what psychoanalysts call the object.

Psychologically speaking, the feeling of being elevated spiritually into the presence of the sublime would then correspond to the confused perception of growth of the mind that occurs when a person finds the right measure of proximity to and distance from the object. Arguably, one could also say: when in relation to it one is at the same time in an *ideal* situation, as opposed to merely physical proximity (another way of referring to the moment of vertigo). But surely in this case the terms proximity and distance translate a dialectic of identity and difference.

Over time, and in its attempt to frame a model for therapeutic action, psychoanalysis has become more and more specialized as a series of reflections on the vicissitudes of this primary relationship between an infant (a child who cannot yet speak), and this other-object or mother, but also a mouthpiece for the Other, that is to say, for culture, sociality, language, the unconscious. The mystery that no aesthetic theory is able to explain, precisely because it is impossible to explain in words something that belongs to the order of sensations, becomes a little less difficult to fathom if we register the co-occurrence of aesthetic form and primary rhythm that establishes original temporality and thought (being). Arguably, what we perceive as an expression of the highest beauty is a "reminiscence" of how a happy conversation with the object first granted us access to the realm of the human[7].

But it is not only "reminiscence", because the process is endlessly repeated. On the one hand, being born is an illusion, since to some extent we always remain imprisoned in the mother's body, albeit, as we have already seen, dilated into the world; on the other hand, we never finish "being born". Thus in art, we seek help each time to be reborn and consequently to mark out firmer boundaries for our ego thanks to the communion with others that makes for aesthetic experience. Indeed, it would be false to think of subjectivity/intersubjectivity as a dichotomy. Rimbaud's[8] famous dictum that "I is another" should be taken literally. If we try to imagine how one becomes a subject, we cannot help thinking of subjectivity (self-awareness) and intersubjectivity (intercorporeality and language) as the two inseparable sides of the same coin or the two poles of a magnet that re-form even if we break it into a thousand fragments. It would be absurd to think that one can come before the other, because from the very outset one necessarily implies the other, both at pre-reflexive and later reflexive stages of the ego's development. What is added at the ontogenesis level is the dizzying acceleration in time due to the fact that, when it is born, the child is already in the human dimension of language and does not have to go through the stages that humanity has been through over thousands of years.

On the basis of what has just been said, the famous Keatsian[9] equation of beauty with truth and the assertion that this is all there is to know and nothing more, becomes something definitive. From today's perspective, the phrase resonates as an anticipation of the problematic closing sentence in Wittgenstein's[10] *Tractatus*. The convergence between the two is interesting. Both Keats and Wittgenstein exhort us to countenance *not* knowing; but this was already the meaning of Tiresias' exhortation to Oedipus not to ask to know the truth about the murder of Laius[11]. Knowing the ultimate roots of being is beyond our grasp. Something more, however, is known if, with Bion, we extend the terms of the equation and equate "truth" with the food that nourishes the mind, that is, the repeated events of ideo-affective attunement that weave the fabric of humanity.

The only way to advance further in our understanding of aesthetic experience would be to espouse a Kantian transcendental aesthetics or perhaps neuroaesthetics. This would, however, entail "regressing" to the meaningless world of the prelinguistic, and we would risk explaining art in a reductionist manner. Equally, it would be tantamount to denying, as perhaps Husserl investigated more than any other, that purely human intersubjectivity, while resting on prehuman, original, instinctual forms of intersubjectivity, is then extended into linguistic intersubjectivity.

Psychoanalysis, on the other hand, starts from what is already human and imaginatively reconstructs how the primary relationship unfolds. Notably, Melanie Klein "created" the world of the newborn and infant, a world that as such did not exist in this way before her, and for which we did not have the words. When the young child suffers frustration, it always experiences it as "deprivation", that is, as active rejection by the beloved object. The "nastiness" of the mother spurs him on in turn to react unconsciously with envious and "murderous" attacks, in the sense of wishing her dead. Among the activities he then undertakes to repair the damaged object, Melanie Klein[12] mentions, construction games in which the child works at "putting one brick on top of another, or making a brick stand upright after it had been knocked down". One is prompted to think of Kiefer's *Heavenly Palaces*. It is clear that just like tenderness, patience, gentleness, love and the experience of being in pleasant contact with the breast, hatred, aggression, and destructiveness are just as essential for coping with the coexistence of extreme and opposite feelings towards the same object of love and for nurturing creativity[13].

If the child cannot deal with the conflict, then he or she will suffer inhibitions and real developmental failures. In the fantasy, cruelty is both suffered and acted out. If, moreover, one reflects on the fact that not only the good breast but also the bad breast is internalized, and that in actual fact we are never completely outside nor completely inside ourselves[14], then, depending on the individual case, the scene of greedy, erotic or destructive impulses may reversibly be one's own body or the body of the other. All of this ultimately chimes in with the experience of the sublime in general, but in some artists and works, as in McQueen and Malani, it takes on a unique cogency and obsessive quality.

Melanie Klein gave depth and perspective, true *concreteness*, to the Freudian intuition of the reality and effectiveness of the inner world. The unconscious is no longer a region of the psyche untouched by civilization, but a theatre teeming with characters, some of which are monstrous and bloody, and above all it is a theatre that never closes. The various characters and the storylines they enact are sources of meaning and significance in the light of which each person constantly reads experience. After all, this is the world of cruel ogres and rescuing and powerful fairies that are recounted in fairy tales and that, as we have seen, we find in contemporary art.

What does it mean then that it is possible to reinvent the concept of sublimation starting from the idea of sublimity? It means that what we see in sublimation is no longer the (unconscious) decision to forgo satisfying a drive, but it is rather the drive to be as much a part of sociality as possible, and thus, if anything, to satisfy it according to standard rules. Bear in mind, however, there is no intersubjectivity, whether prerifiexive or dialogical, that does not rest on the ground of the transcendental proto-intersubjectivity of the animal and the sexual community of instincts. There is therefore no necessary dichotomy between drive and sociality.

Sublimation does not imply the definitive eschewal of sexual gratification, which can be said to be as liberating as it is repressive. By reconnecting with wider sociality, ideally, it represents an attempt by the subject to enhance its capacity to love both spiritually and physically, and not the other way around. If we come up against constant blockages that thwart this capacity, it is because the subject is unsuccessful in achieving its goal, and rather experiences yet further rejection.

Thinking of sublimation in these terms makes it possible to dispel some of the reservations that weigh down the concept: how to differentiate small, everyday acts of sublimation from large, successful ones; how to explain by the obscure mechanism whereby drive energy is diverted; wherein lies the difference between those who succeed in "sublimating" by creating something for everyone and those who fail to do so.

The aesthetics of the sublime, which can look back on a very sophisticated theoretical history in speculative thought, when it produces concrete artistic realizations, contributes to a rethinking of sublimation with its productive ambiguity of images, with the sensoriality of emotions. What we gain from this operation is not only an intellectual understanding, but also an understanding from within (immediate, affective, libidinal), which for this reason can be considered both more complete and truer. One could go so far as to say that any aesthetic experience theorizes – both thematically in the abstract and experientially in the affective body – the birth of the psyche from the dialectical interrelationship between (proto-)subjectivity and (proto-)intersubjectivity.

Notes

1 See S. Freud, 1930, *Civilization and Its Discontents*, cit., p. 130, in footnote.
2 B. Newman, "The Sublime is Now", in *Selected Writings and Interviews*, 1990, 170–173, edited by J. P. O'Neill, University of California Press, Berkeley and Los Angeles, 1992.
3 See M.-L. Ryan, 2001, *Narrative as Virtual Reality: Immersion and Interactivity in Literature and Electronic Media*, Baltimore, MD, Johns Hopkins UP, 2003.
4 See J. Derrida, *The Truth in Painting*, transl. by G. Bennington and I. McLeod, The University of Chicago Press, Chicago, 1987.
5 R. Barthes, *The Pleasure of the Text*, cited, p. 37.
6 J.-B. Pontalis, "Il á été rêvé", in A. Mazzarella and J. Risset, eds., *Scene del sogno*. It. tr by A. dell'Armi, pp. 11–24, Artemide, Roma 2003.
7 See W. R. Bion, *Transformations,* Karnac, London, 1965, p. 106, footnote, for the analogy between the encounter of "preconception" as a kind of innate predisposition to "encounter" a certain object or "realization" and the "the concept of Platonic forms of which the personalityis 'reminded' by contact with a real object."

8 A. Rimbaud, (1871). *A Season in Hell and Illuminations*, transl. B. Mathieu. Boa Editions, Rochester, NY, 1991, p. 85.

9 J. Keats, "Ode on a Grecian Urn": "Beauty is truth, truth beauty", – that is all / Ye know on earth", https://en.wikipedia.org/wiki/Ode_on_a_Grecian_Urn (accessed on Dec. 5th, 2022).

10 L. Wittgenstein, 1921, *Tractatus Logico-Philosophicus*, transl. by D. F. Pears & B. F. McGuinnes, Routledge, London, 1974, p. 89: "What we cannot speak about we must pass over in silence".

11 For Bion, the central conflict of the human being is not between Oedipus and Laius, but between Oedipus and Tiresias, that is, between the desire to know and the inaccessibility of truth (in his terminology jargon: between K and minus-K).

12 M. Klein, 1936, *On the Bringing up of Children* [1939], Routledge, London, 2001, p. 38.

13 See D. W. Winnicott, (1975) "Hate in the Countertransference" [1947]. *Through Paediatrics to Psycho-Analysis* 100:194–203.

14 See J. P. Sartre, *The Transcendence of the Ego: A Sketch for a Phenomenological Description*, 1936, transl. by A. Brown, Routledge, London, 2004, p. 1: "the Ego is neither formally nor materially *in* consciousness: it is outside, in the world; it is a being *in the world*, like the Ego of another".

12

THE ABJECT BODY

Blood is both visible and invisible. We feel it as it courses pulsating, pressing, ebbing, and flowing. We sense the colour changes it produces in the skin, but we never see it directly. Unless, that is, we have an open wound. Yet we speak of blood as the element that more than any other coincides with our identity. Blood is the image par excellence of our inner life and the drives that animate it. In the body, as McQueen says, there is always a layer of blood under the skin. Similarly, in the sublime blood always lies "under the skin" of landscapes that are ultimately always anthropomorphized and therefore steeped in human emotions. It is understandable why in his last unfinished work, *The Visible and the Invisible*, Merleau-Ponty[1] called "flesh" the true grain of life.

When it comes down to it, what does the art system do other than insist on saying "look… and look again…"? The special perceptual regime it establishes invites us to go beyond the surface to see the blood or flesh of the world. It animates this regime with a tendency to transpose all things. If there is a difference between the merely beautiful and the sublime, it lies in the fact that in the actual artistic gesture, both in form and content, the sublime continues to articulate an aesthetic. The sublime reveals that beneath the visible of nature, there is the invisible of nothingness; not only nothingness as the concrete end of existence, but the immanence of nothingness in language, in the now and in the self, and thus in all things[2]. In this way, he also reveals to us that which *cannot* be seen but which works away to structure the experience even of something which is *simply* beautiful or pleasurable.

As we move from Serra's installation to Kiefer's, the thematic complexity of the work grows, and the number of explicit references

 DOI: 10.4324/9781003478904-12

becomes encyclopaedic. The path we have outlined resembles a kind of progression that recounts the gradual entry of animal-man into the world of the symbolic, made up initially of sensory scans, but going on to include the rules and laws consubstantial to language. This is why ultimately there is not much to say about Serra. Experience is reduced to the essentiality of muscular and visceral sensations of movement and sense impressions. Serra and Kapoor proceed "by subtraction" because their goal is to lay bare the "sensitive" side of subjectivity, the habitual patterns that give the ego the illusion of compactness and coherence, and not so much the more intellectual side. The *sensitive* ventricle of the ego is the one that pulsates from the beginning of life; the rational-abstract one also pulsates from birth, but it is eccentric because it is in the o/Other.

It is as if the *before* of the word situated us in the purely intercorporeal and kinesthetic dimension of the original constitution of subjectivity. To this ever-present dimension are gradually added others that are more and more sophisticated in terms of culture and sociality. The process of subjectivation, in other words the attainment of sufficient "remoteness", however, involves a succession of several stages. The process is radically social. Birth must be negotiated with the Other, but when playing the first hand it is the Other who holds all the cards.

The reality is that the mother herself gives rise in the newborn to the pain she promises to soothe. Having given birth to the child, she is at the root of this essentially "dissociated" emotional situation. In a mirror image of this, envy and gratitude, or rather their affective precursors, get constantly mixed up in the child. What McQueen does particularly well is to portray the conflict that arises between these two aspects when they are still irreconcilable: on the one hand, the pain (and the hatred that arises from it), and on the other hand, the pleasure that results from relieving it. In her icy being, the woman reduced to a mannequin, or rather disguised as a mannequin, expresses the power to subjugate. The streaks of blood show both that she is the object of innumerable acts of vengeance and that the aggressions also render visible what is invisible in her internal landscape.

Transposed from the body as landscape to the body as mother, the dramatic thrust already present in such sentimental views of the sublime reaches its acme. The struggle to be born is inescapable in the attempt to attain life. Paraphrasing the Mad Hatter from *Alice in Wonderland*, we could say that it is always "birth-time", the hour of birth. Melanie Klein and Julia Kristeva are the best at telling us what the struggle is. It is the struggle to make the maternal body abject and thus build a safe enough home[3] for the self.

Already in the Platonic myth of the symposium, what is important is the lacerating rift that is produced in the "flesh" of the world. Oozing from the irreparable original wound comes desire (itself a form of pain) and jouissance; ever since then they have been inseparable twins, we now call eros or sexuality. Being attracted to the object is both a blessing in life and the curse of the excruciating feeling of incompleteness that always accompanies it.

Taking inspiration from Hegel, Lacan[4], in *The Function and Field of Speech and Language in Psychoanalysis*, writes that "the symbol first manifests itself as the killing of the thing, and this death results in the endless perpetuation of the subject's desire"—although one could argue that it is impossible to kill something one cannot get at and which literally does not "exist". It would be more correct to say that, rather than killing it, one gives it life; or rather that one gives it life by killing it. As we know, Hegel himself asserts that being is nothingness. What does this mean? That the *negative* is part of us right down to the very deepest fibre of our being, deeper by far than we would be willing to admit according to the common sense that guides us in our everyday affairs. "Being" means existing as human beings, that is, animals endowed with language. But language is nothing other than the exercise we engage in all the time, even when we think we are alone, as we play hide-and-seek with nothingness so as to bring something into existence. We can only attain self-awareness if linguistic signs we admit to partially having lost the real, that is, to transforming it into nothingness ("re-removing" it), a real that, however, without this operation, would not exist for us at all. Without language, we would no longer exist as subjects and nothing would stand in front of us as objects.

Another way of describing this struggle to exist by disentangling ourselves from the real is to say that we must make it abject. This term refers to the process of separating oneself from something that until recently had been part of one's body and doing so with a certain quantum of inevitable violence. An example of this is the lock of hair that McQueen used as a label for his clothes. This applies even more so to vomit, urine, faeces, nails, mucus, saliva, sweat, pus, blood, etc. These are all elements that force us to realize that the body (the house) is made up of boundaries between inside and outside, but that these boundaries can be transcended and are therefore neither absolute nor inviolable. Could it be that this is because they are immediately charged with something deadly?

Disgust for the bodily fragment that is now dead is a mirroring no longer in the Other as an containing and transforming object, but in a double, and as such a harbinger of death. It is a feeling of "depersonalization" not suffered directly in the body that is not yet one's own, but displaced into minimal emanations that are no longer part of it. In their disquieting concreteness, the fragments of skin, the cut or fallen hair, and the bodily fluids suggest the psychic fragmentation that occurs when there is no longer the mirror of the Other to grant the subject access to the symbolic and keep him there. To rid himself of these sensations, he must exclude the abject, protect himself from its infection, and reinstate the limits of the body. The abject is in fact the disappearance of the Other as symbolic and its resurfacing instead as something threateningly real.

Yet death, the abject by definition, gives meaning to life. As the poet Chandra Livia Candiani says, "It is important not to forget that there is death. I make all my choices in the light of death. I have no time to waste"[5]. It is also, as in Tolstoy[6], the last defence against pain. Freud[7] explained that without the feeling of transience there would be no aesthetic experience. This means that boundaries must not be sealed but kept porous. If necessary, the caesura must become permeable. A contact barrier regulates the subject's dealings with the abject by placing it at a certain distance. This is what art does when it disposes its various protective frames. We need the abject, but to enjoy it we must wear the protective glasses of aesthetic form.

The maternal body, which is originally experienced as part of one's own body, is the abject with a capital "A". It is the very prototype of all the abject elements listed above. It is transformed into Kubin's hideous crustacean-spider. But it is precisely the mother who triggers the process whereby first the physical and then the moral filth becomes abject for the infant. We rediscover that the abject (what we see as corrupt, filthy, execrable, disgusting, despicable, filthy, repugnant; but also morally vile, mean, cowardly, dishonest, dastardly, obscene, ungodly, etc.) cannot be erased, as it is the other side of the coin of life (which we see as whole, noble, honest, human, pure, probable, modest, honoured, meritorious, etc.).

Julia Kristeva's concept of abjection recasts Freud's[8] notion of the uncanny in a new context and draws out its full heuristic potential.

Both are phenomena of the return of the repressed, the unconscious psychic mechanism that serves to ward off a disturbing stimulus. But while the disturbing is linked to secondary repression, which in the first instance depends on the subject's superego, the abject is linked to primary repression[9], which in an infant depends on a superego that is not its own, as it cannot yet exist, but exclusively on that of the object. In this way, unlike the concept of the uncanny, the abject has the merit of exalting even more the intersubjective essence of the process and its pre-reflexive and inter-corporeal (semiotic) dimension, albeit in relation to the vicissitudes of access to the symbolic.

In fact, the symbolic has always been there present, in the head and the body of the mother[10]. This is why a total rejection of the mother's body, as occurs in certain severe states of infantile autism, can make it impossible for the child to enter the human world of language, in the same way as, in Freudian psychoanalysis, if the action of repression, whether primary or secondary, were prevented, the psyche could not be formed. Like repression, the abject has the function of tracing the contours of the self and thus of constituting it; opposed to it but coinciding with it is in fact the "limit" represented by the boundaries of the self.

This is why, in order to get a sense of limits, people follow rituals throughout their lives that bring them to come into contact with the abject without being overwhelmed by it. Whether we are talking about the stage in the theatre or the frame around a painting, the cinema screen, or the expiry date on a yoghurt pot, the point is always to enter into clearly delimited contact with the abject. The attraction, but also the love that the subject feels for the abject (or the uncanny), arises from the obscure awareness that it contributes to confirming him as subject; that it is one of the two terms (the other is its opposite, the non-abject) whose dialectical relationship produces the "spiritual" elevation of the subject. It goes without saying that the terms attraction and love are confusing here because they presuppose an I that in the infant's situation has yet to come into being. Nonetheless, I use these terms to indicate what I see as their most distant roots. They are rooted in a field of psychic tensions which, while presupposing the Other, first and foremost materializes in the flesh as bodily co-intentionality.

To gaze upon the abject is like watching the blood flowing under one's skin and recognizing its vital function. The matrix of the abject is found in Freud's description of how disgust for faeces arises in the child, which in turn precedes the sense of shame and morality as agents of psychic repression and guarantors of the prohibition of incest. Disgust, Freud writes, "interferes with the libidinal over-valuation of the sexual object but can in turn be overridden by libido"[11]. When the insertion of the merely real of the abject into the symbolic succeeds, then we have the sublimation of the semiotic into language, that is, access to the experience of the transitional object described by Winnicott. The concept of the abject thus makes us realize that sublimation is not only the socially determined refinement of language concepts, but also a process of dematerialization of the anatomical body and its transposition into the lived body.

In short, the abject functions as the friction that allows one to gain traction on the ground, or as the hard object from which the autistic child derives a bodily feeling of self-delimitation. In this view, if there is any pathology it is brought about by the collapse of the dialectic between the abject as rejection and the abject as a sense of limit. For example, to spit on something is to express the highest possible rejection, i.e. to mortify ("kill"). The fact is that the subject who uses saliva as an abject object, in doing so necessarily identifies disturbingly with this former object of his. Metonymically, the abject object reminds him that he himself in all his being is an abject object, and that he will become such most manifestly at death.

The abject has an intermediate, transitive, ambiguous dimension, on a par with that of words. The word itself is potentially an abject object, that is, an object that becomes alienated as soon as it is detached from the body that uttered it – as happens when we sometimes let slip something we immediately regret or feel ashamed of. At the very instant it is uttered, any word becomes an uncanny mix of familiarity and strangeness. On the one hand, it confirms identity, and on the other, it forces identity into a state of crisis, which may lead to regression or growth. Obviously, the symbolic matrix that generates the abject cannot belong to the infant from birth; it does belong, however, to the field of the relationship with the object because it is the latter that guarantees its presence. At birth, the violence of what is abject, i.e. thrown away, is the same violence as "interpretation"[12]. The abject is ultimately the symbolic equivalent of Ernst's reel and of any phonetic opposition[13]. To return one last time to Freud's brilliant reflections on the *fort/da* game, one could argue that what Ernst throws away is not just the reel as a symbolic substitute for the mother, but himself, or rather his own flesh, and that he then takes it back in a "spiritualized" form as an abstraction of his own body-as-real, and thus as body-symbol, as self or lived body. In short, the Word becomes flesh or the flesh receives the Word.

In conclusion, Kristeva's concept of abjection, more "intersubjective" than how the author herself presents it to us, inscribes the Freudian concept of the uncanny in an extremely rich dimension of current psychoanalytic research. The moment of vertigo that the feeling of the uncanny marks in the evolution of the psyche is equivalent to the essential instability of the ego and the fluidity of the body. It is due to the fact that by subject we must mean a fabric made of the interwoven threads of the weft of subjectivity (difference) and the warp of intersubjectivity (identity). There are social rules that draw a geography that is permitted and one that is prohibited to bodies, to certain bodies, or to certain bodies in particular conditions. It is clear that bodies are as much material as they are socially constructed, *written*, scrutinized, and regulated.

That the body is a continuously written text becomes very clear when this process fails to achieve its purpose. For example, Kelly Fuery[14] has analyzed the TV miniseries *Sharp Objects* in the light of Bion's concept of "bizarre object"[15]. One of the characters, Camilla, hallucinates words written as scars on bodies or objects. The idea is that when inter-subjective ties diminish (the degree of consensuality, that which makes trauma unthinkable) she veers towards concrete thought. Words then solidify and become things. The narrative device is intriguing. It is as if at the moment when the subject turns away from the social community or language as the "house of being"[16] she is forced to realize the fiction of things and the world (because she can only see them as a thinking being and thus as subject to the God-language). In actual fact, this is precisely what Camille *cannot* do. The fiction that sustains our naive realism, i.e. the fiction that is not perceived in the same way as the process of digestion is not perceived when it does not cause problems, is overturned in the madness of the person who unmasks and denounces this fiction, but in doing so loses her own sense of reality and is no longer believed.

Language makes an artificial cut between the self and the body-as-thing and between words and things. Whenever we have the sensation that this hiatus is beginning to narrow and even tends towards zero, we feel the thrill of becoming one with the whole again, of losing ourselves in the real of mere matter and undifferentiation; but at the same time, we are also one with the real that stands out in the human community. In short, the aesthetic experience is vertiginous because it pulls in two opposing directions (such as *to* or *from* the object), and joy is pain and pain joy. We could try to distinguish between those drives that appear to us to correspond to a life drive and those that correspond more to a death drive. The fact is, however, they are like the different sides of a Moebius strip. They follow one another but continuously. They are at the same time life drives and death drives, and the subject can only stand in *between* them. Poetry and art in general are the secular forms in which this antagonistic solidarity between opposing impulses, both in search of existence, is performed.

Poetry tends to dissolve meaning into sense, semantics into the semiotic, and the visual into the musical, but at the same time it generates a surplus of meaning. Exposure to the abject but under safe conditions. By regressing into the opacity of meaning, the subject has the opportunity to lean over the abyss of the real. And this gives meaning to existence, as Heidegger recognized so well with his theme of authenticity (*Eigentlichkeit*, which literally means "self-mastery"[17]). In a dialogue between Freud and Heidegger[18], the expression "death drive" (*pulsione di morte*) could be understood as a subjective genitive; as if to say that it is the prospect of death that generates the drive to live. As in the technique of psychoanalysis, it is a functional regression that actually serves the thrust towards progress. This is what makes for a surplus of meaning. But one should not deceive oneself. The category of aesthetics does not eschew universality; simply enough, instead of operating like reason via abstraction; it makes sensation universal by starting from what is less universal, that is, from concrete experience.

What artists do is to expand the boundaries of the abject and reclaim new territories where the seedling of the self can be planted and grown. There is a constant move to subvert already established disciplinary systems and to annex new areas of the abject (of the negative or "foreign") to the civilization of the self. This makes it stronger and more effective. In essence, when reflected in the mirror of the abject, what the uncanny speaks to us about is the struggle between the spectre of death and the possibility of authentic existence. The former comes back to threaten the subject whenever the presence of the object becomes imminent (Lacan or *Psycho*); the latter arises out of being able to gain a perspective, a certain distance or remoteness from it (this is the great construction site that enlists the energies of adolescents, but also others). Clearly, when it comes to the concept of the sublime, what is at stake is nothing less than our conception of what is human and what constitutes the essence of the practice of treating psychic suffering inaugurated by Freud: what if not the art of welcoming unexpected guests into one's home?

Notes

1 M. Merleau-Ponty, 1964, *The Visible and the Invisible*, cited.

2 G. W. F. Hegel, *The Science of Logic*, transl. by G. Di Giovanni, Cambridge University Press, Cambridge, 2010, pp. 59–60: "*Pure being and pure nothing are therefore the same.* The truth is neither being nor nothing, but rather that being has passed over into nothing and nothing into being – 'has passed over,' not passes over. But the truth is just as much that they are not without distinction; it is rather that *they are not the same*, that they are absolutely distinct yet equally unseparated and inseparable, and that *each* immediately *vanishes in its opposite*. Their truth is therefore this *movement* of the immediate vanishing of the one into the other: *becoming*, a movement in which the two are distinguished, but by a distinction which has just as immediately dissolved itself".

3 On the concept of home, see G. Civitarese and S. Boffito, "Intime stanze. La casa della psicoanalisi", in *Le case dell'uomo. Abitare il mondo*, pp. 29–42, Utet, Turin 2016. See also S. Petrosino, *Lo spirito della casa. Ospitalità, intimità e giustizia*, cit., pp. 46–47: "In walking through that room, in opening that window, in re-dressing that bed and that kitchen, the subject is invested with memories, sensations, feelings, and so, without having properly decided to do so, he finds himself revising, reliving and rethinking, imagining and fantasizing, as if he is taken in by a stream of emotions and words that reveals to him how that room and that window, that bed and that kitchen were never mere objects at his disposal or mere spaces to be occupied, being rather his own place, 'his own home' without property". Lastly, see J. Derrida, 1997, *Adieu to Emmanuel Levinas*, transl. by P.-A Brault and M. Naas, Stanford: Stanford University Press, 1999, p. 41–42: "the one who welcomes the invited or received *hôte* (the guest), the welcoming *hôte* who considers himself the owner of the place, is in truth a *hôte* received in his own home. He receives the hospitality that he offers in his own home [...] The one who invites is invited by the one whom he invites".

4 J. Lacan, "The Function and Field of Speech and Language in Psychoanalysis", 1966, pp. 197–268, in *Écrits,* transl. by B. Fink, W. W. Norton & Company, New York, 2006, p. 262.

5 A. Briganti, "Chandra Livia Candiani: 'Si medita a occhi chiusi per imparare ad aprirli'", *La Repubblica* 20-1-2019. https://ricerca.repubblica.it/

repubblica/archivio/repubblica/2019/01/20/chandra-livia-candiani-si-medita-a-occhi-chiusi-aprirliMilano12.html?ref=search

6 L. Tolstoy, *Anna Karenina*, transl. by N. Haskell Dole, Thomas Y. Crowell & Company, New York, 1899, p. 347, https://archive.org/details/annakareninatols00tolsiala/page/n673/mode/2up?q=nikolay (accessed Dec. 6th, 2022): "Evidently there was accomplishing in him that revolution whereby he would be induced to look on death as a consummation of his desires, even as a joy. Hitherto, every individual desire called forth by suffering or privation, as by hunger, weariness, thirst, was satisfied by some bodily exercise producing pleasure; but now privation and suffering got no relief and any attempt at relieving them caused new suffering. And so all his desires were concentrated on one thing,—the wish to be delivered from all his woes and the very source of his woes, from his body. But he had no words to express this thought, and he continued out of habit to ask for what once gave him comfort, but could no longer satisfy him".

7 See S. Freud, "On Transience", Freud, S. (1916 [1915]). The Standard Edition of the Complete Psychological Works of Sigmund Freud 14:303–307. The essay is a little gem that can be interpreted in many different ways. For example, it can be seen not only in the context of the question of beauty, but also in the Oedipal competition between Freud, now an old man, and Rilke, the young but already established poet, over Lou Andreas Salomé, the mutual friend who can be recognised as the third character going on the walk.

8 S. Freud, The "Uncanny". The Standard Edition of the Complete Psychological Works of Sigmund Freud 17:217–256, 1919.

9 In Freud this remains a rather obscure concept. We can think of it as a mode through which by semiotic means culture, mediated by the object, begins to install the norm in the infant's body.

10 See A. J. Greimas, *Structural Semantics: An Attempt at a Method*, 1966, transl. by D. McDowell, R. Schleifer, and A. Velie, University of Nebraska Press, Lincoln, 1983, p. 6: "One is naïvely surprised when one starts to reflect upon the situation of man, who, from morning to evening and from birth to death, is literally assailed by significations challenging him from everywhere, by messages reaching him at every moment and in all forms. How naïve—in the nonscientific sense of the word—the pretensions of some literary movements appear, wishing to establish an aesthetics of nonsignification".

11 See S. Freud, *Three Essays on the Theory of Sexuality* (1905). The Standard Edition of the Complete Psychological Works of Sigmund Freud 7:123–246, 1905, p. 152.

12 See P. Aulagnier, *The Violence of Interpretation: From Pictogram to Statement*, 1975, transl. by A. Sheridan, Routledge, London, 2001.

13 See R. Chemama, B. Vandermersch, *Dizionario di psicoanalisi*, 1998, It. tr. by C. Albarello, L. Burzotta, M. Drazien. C. Fanelli, M. Fiumanò, J. Jerkov, S. Paparello, J. Venneman, Gremese, 2004, p. 143: at its zero degree it is already the "oppositional link of two syllables of language with the repetition of the loss and the appearance of the desired object, pleasure and pain, that can define enjoyment". But then can we not see in this play of syllables a pure rhythm expressed in a kind of song? And is rhythm not the prime vehicle of a (so to speak) musical or semiotic sense that precedes the meaning of the word? In the interpretation that Sophie, little Ernst's mother, gives of what starts out as the pure play of syllables we see this transformation that is always on the point of being completed, but also of unravelling, and the inevitably transindividual or intersubjective dimension (the thread, the bond) in which only it can happen. If we did not take into account the role of the presence of others and of language even in its purely rhythmic component, we would not understand how concepts are formed or how the ability to think develops. Hence the usefulness of taking music as a model. It is language that is a-semantic but not a-symbolic. It is perhaps the means of expression that exerts the greatest power on our emotional states. Might this be because it is pure temporality? Or because, when it resonates with the melody of our being, it realigns us with time? Or because it gives us a semiotic form that repairs the defects of our time? But then shouldn't we pay more attention to the intersubjective and aesthetic dimension in which subjectivity is constructed? Shouldn't we consider the body more and give more importance to sense (procedural/implicit/corporeal 'sense') and less to conceptual/linguistic/explicit meaning? In the words of G. Deleuze, F. Guattari, *A Thousand Plateaus: Capitalism and Schizophrenia* [1980], transl. by B. Massumi, University of Minnesota Press, Minneapolis, 1987, p. 299: "What does music deal with, what is the content indissociable from sound expression? It is hard to say, but it is something: a child dies, a child plays, a woman is born, a woman dies, a bird arrives, a bird flies off. We wish to say that these are not accidental themes in music (even if it is possible to multiply examples), much less imitative exercises; they are something essential. Why a child, a woman, a bird? It is because musical expression is inseparable from a becoming-woman, a becoming-child, a becoming-animal that constitute its content".

14 K. Fuery, "Transformation, Hallucination and Memory as Bizarre (Sharp) Object", paper read at the conference *Film in Focus. Psychoanalysis and Contemporary Cinema*, London, July 21 2019.

15 For the definition of "bizarre object", see W. R. Bion, *Second Thoughts: Selected Papers on Psycho-Analysis*, Heineman, London, 1967. For a psychotic patient, bizarre objects are expelled ego particles or personality

fragments that encapsulate or are encapsulated in concretely existing objects. In the unconscious fantasy such objects lead independent lives.

16 M. Heidegger, *Pathmarks*, 1947, edited by W. McNeill, Cambridge University Press, Cambridge, 1988, p. 239.

17 On this concept, see J.-J- Koo, "Heidegger's Underdeveloped Conception of the Undistinguishedness (*Indifferenz*) of Everyday Human Existence", in H. B. Schmid and G. Thonauser, eds., *From Conventionalism to Social Authenticity. Heidegger's Anyone and Contemporary Social Theory*, pp. 53–78, 2017, where the author distinguishes between three possible fates for the individual: there are those who live their whole lives quietly in the conformity of the social group to which they belong, a bit like a sleepwalker (*Indifferenz/undistinguishedness*); those who experience the shock of distress and manage to escape from indistinction (*Eigentlichkeit/ownedness*); finally, those who, having had the opportunity, opt for inauthenticity (*Uneigentlichkeit/unownedness*), in order to escape from the feeling of distress.

18 See also G. Berto's *Freud, Heidegger, Lo spaesamento*, Bompiani, Milan 2002.

13

OH LIFE, BEGUN IN A BLOODY FLOW[1]

If it is true that a psychoanalytic reading of the sublime makes sense, then it follows that there is no justification for too sharp a distinction between "simple" beauty and the sublime. I cannot see why there should be a difference not simply of degree but also of kind. Quite plainly, in my view, the sublime merely exhibits the essential structure of aesthetic experience but on a much larger scale than "pleasurable" beauty. Any sensation of the beautiful, no matter how minimal or fleeting, *always* reminds us of the transience of all things and thus always implies some kind of grief work. The feelings evoked by the beautiful and the sublime are connected in some way or another to an elegy to life and the world, on the one hand, and to the horror of the unrepresentable quality of death on the other hand. The aesthetic experience is thus inevitably imbued with nostalgia, in other words, the pain of remembering, and "leth-algia", i.e. the pain of *not* being able to remember. It arises out of the pain-filled desire to return to the places of one's birth (what Freud refers to as the first "Heim"), or out of no longer knowing where they are.

As Byung-Chul Han[2] says: "The beautiful and the sublime have the same origin. Instead of opposing the sublime to the beautiful, one should [...] undo the separation of the beautiful and the sublime". And then again to quote Lyotard[3]:

> *Delight*, or the negative pleasure which in contradictory, almost neurotic fashion, characterizes the feeling of the sublime, arises from the removal of the threat of pain. Certain 'objects' and certain 'sensations' are pregnant with a threat to our self-preservation, and Burke refers to that threat as *terror*: shadows, solitude, silence, and approach of death may be 'terrible' in that they announce that

DOI: 10.4324/9781003478904-13

the gaze, the other, language or life will soon be extinguished. One feels that it is possible that soon nothing more will take place. What is sublime is the feeling that something will happen, despite everything' within this threatening void, that something will take 'place' and will announce that everything is not over. That place is mere 'here', the most minimal occurrence

I agree, although I would add that it is not only a *here* but also a *now*. In our modern and contemporary times, abstract art also expresses the sublime – for example, the pure lines, the angles of certain geometric shapes – because they evoke the chaos of creation. From this point of view, the obscurity at issue in the contemporary sublime is merely an allusion to the as-if quality of thought on the one hand, and a metaphysics of the invisible intentions of the object on the other hand. It is an artificial reading to claim, as Newman[4] does, that modern art is void of sublime content. It is there even when it consists only of the geometric perfection of the white surface and the right angle, as in Mondrian, or pure chromaticism, as in Rothko – for obvious reasons, an artist whose canvases have been associated with the concept of "numinous". In their case, too, there is grandiosity, but it is a "negative" grandiosity. The infinitesimal is just as vast as the Kantian mathematical sublime. That is why a simple interweaving of lines can conceal an abyss.

In other cases, an artist may use the technique of blowing some infinitely small element out of proportion. As in Kapoor's *Symphony for a Beloved Sun*, which does not proceed directly towards the grandiose, but towards the infinitely microscopic grain of matter (*the infinitesimal*) and only then seeks to make it visible, magnified out of all proportion. This is, for instance, what is intimated by Liu Wei's installation Microworld (2018; Fig. 13.1).

Standing around in a shrine the size of a large room are mysterious spheres and other rounded shapes that are absolutely out of proportion, intended as representations of the prime elements of matter, somewhat like a comic strip designed to illustrate Democritean theories, atoms and molecules, the infinite variety of the minimal, indivisible and normally imperceptible particles of which matter is made. In inverse proportion, it is the spectator who shrinks, and who is denied access to the objects of this strange universe by a large transparent wall. This deconstructive operation reveals that behind the visible perception there is the "sensible" of temporality and thus

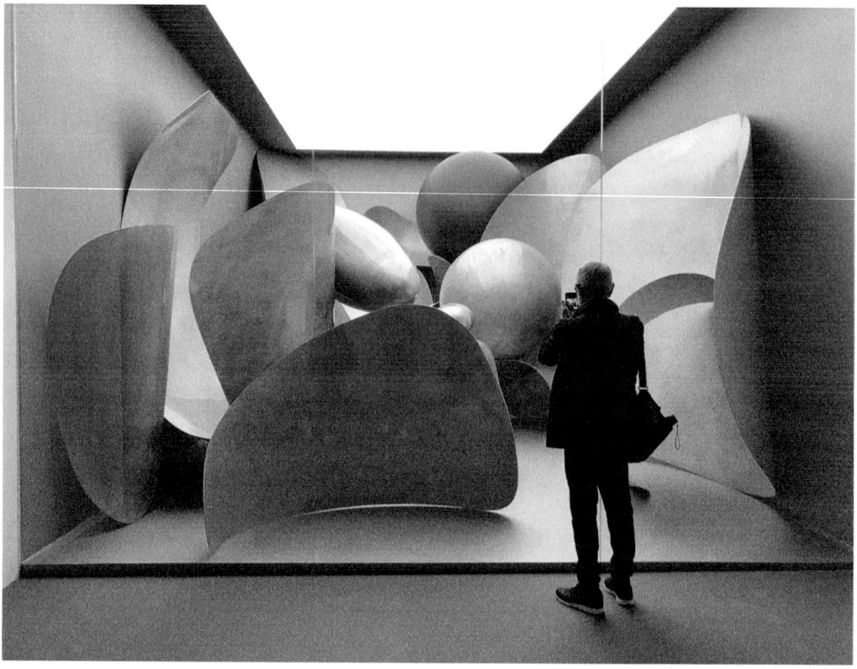

Fig. 13.1 Liu Wei, *Microworld*, 2018. Installation at the 58th Venice Biennale of Visual Arts *May You Live in Interesting Times.* | Photo: Eleonora Zamparutti for © 2019 ARTE.it

the succession of time-points. The yearning for spiritual elevation expressed in the sublime is merely reversed. The goal, though, is identical: to rise up to the level of the gaze of the object and achieve the *ék-stasis* of recognition. At its origin, however, recognition is never conscious, dialogical, and rational, but rather, rhythm, time, *at-one-ment*, "the wonderful surprise, the wonder that there should be something rather than nothing"[5]. In essence, this is the function of art: each time it reinstates the psyche in the body and gives the body back to the psyche.

So not only overt, full-blown grandeur, but also that which manifests through subtraction, empty. Even the infinitely small makes the invisible visible; it's just that it is a negative theophany. Surely what even simple beauty institutes is a heightened awareness of the *here* and *now*. Indeed, what we now know is that the categories of space and time are not *a priori*, as Kant claims, but the outcome of a "mortal" struggle for psychic birth.

Again, in order to effectively account for this, all we have is Melanie Klein's expressionist language, or the *pàthos* that pervades the Hegelian myth of the struggle for recognition in the relationship between lord and servant. Now, what is important to grasp here is that the struggle is between the nascent subject and the maternal body. It is a struggle that begins in the flow of blood, as we read in a line by Emily Dickinson, echoes of which resonate in Sappho's equally sublime phrase "a subtle fire runs through me", or in Hans Castorp's dream in Thomas Mann's[6] *Magic Mountain*, a terrible interpretative variant of Kubin's "spider" in *The Hour of Birth*:

> Two grey old women, witchlike, with hanging breasts and dugs of finger-length, were busy there, between flaming braziers, most horribly. They were dismembering a child. In dreadful silence they tore it apart with their bare hands—Hans Castorp saw the bright hair blood-smeared—and cracked the tender bones between their jaws, their dreadful lips dripped blood. An icy coldness held him. He would have covered his eyes and fled, but could not. They at their gory business had already seen him, they shook their reeking fists and and uttered curses—soundlessly, most vilely, with the last obscenity, and in the dialect of Hans Castorp's native Hamburg.

What runs through the works we have briefly touched upon so far is the obsession with blood. Serra's labyrinth summons up the palace of Knossos and Kafka's *The Lair*, Malani's irresistible nightmare the human sacrifices of *Heart of Darkness*, McQueen's[7] necrophilic world the sadomasochistic perversion and its sometimes bloody rituals, Kapoor's *beloved/bloody sun/son* the violence that can reign in a post-apocalyptic world. The wound inflicted on the female body is reminiscent of the "cutting" of the mother's body to see the blood of her true intentions flowing under the skin (*in the mind*), in order to cut oneself away, and at the same time *not* to be cut away. The cut is that of birth and the umbilical cord, but also of that which is reborn in the wrenching feeling of desire. In the act of being uttered, each word sanctions the cut and repeats anew its effect of simultaneously generating pleasure and pain.

The scrap of matter that is inexorably lost during the process of ego construction, which then amounts in all respects to access to language, is then first and foremost the materiality of the mother's body. The abjectification of the mother's body is but the first stage in the process whereby language enables one to identify oneself by "abstracting" oneself from reality. Even long before any "subjective" determination, our animality resides in our undifferentiated relationship with the mother's body; in the experience – which can only be theorized a posteriori, but which perhaps resides as an embodied memory – of a state of our being constituted by an indistinct flow of sensations. The physical separation from this materiality which Julia Kristeva describes with the concept of abjection precedes the psychic one. The latter only follows when the former can be thought of. Physical detachment is the prototype of the relative detachment from things that are realized in the process of symbolization through language[8].

Ascent, which is ascent to thought, is a question of freeing oneself from entanglement with the mother's body. In other words, the multiple relational experiences with the primary object sediment become deposited within pre-symbolic and symbolic categories. This corresponds to the idea (again we owe it to Kristeva, although ultimately it derives from Klein) that imaginary matricide lies at the origin of the symbol[9]. Thus, we sometimes hear delusional (but from the point of view of the inner world absolutely "true") accounts by patients who accuse their mothers of having sucked out all their vital energy and who spend their entire lives in a vain attempt to steer clear of this curse. Their experience is not one of living but living-*against*, in which they must constantly repeat an enormous effort to reanimate themselves. Present, concrete life disappears, remaining a mere semblance against the hallucinatory vividness of the object's imminence.

As psychopathology has taught us, the outcome of the struggle to exist is not a foregone conclusion. Through the aesthetics of the sublime, we discover that there is something "heroic" rather than self-evident about representation. To realize this, one only has to listen to patients who go through a crisis in the ability to represent; for example, patients who complain of bodily transformation symptoms that psychiatry labels depersonalization. They readily fall into states of panic, in which they feel their body as if it were collapsing and liquefying. They feel clumsy in their movements, as if their spontaneous motility has broken down. Lacking the automatism of habits, they then force themselves to compensate for the deficit by means of painful efforts of thought. They complain that they no longer have a body, that they are transparent in the eyes of others. They feel they have been reduced to shadows or that they are made of glass. They say that every time they fail to perform a movement that they used to be able to do without even thinking about it, they plunge into total despondency. The fact is that when their body falters, trembles or is gripped by vertigo, it is as if they are forced to direct their gaze at the negative, at absence, at death, at the nothingness that is constitutive of being.

We could liken the obsessive component of checking and scrutinizing that is present in states of depersonalization to rituals for warding off dangers. Perhaps this is the key to grasping its meaning. It is like the experience of escaping a grave danger and the disbelief your body feels at being alive. When one "touches" the body – even just a cursory examination of it or giving it a thought – it is as if the subject imagines magically erasing the disturbing thought of having a decomposing body. In any superstitious gesture, it is enough to touch an object (an "object") made of wood or iron to ward off evil, and one is reassured with regard to the phobic element. As in the case of gestures dictated by superstition, one is always dealing with another an Other from whom one expects protection against the possibility of encountering death. On the level of fantasy, such an eventuality is never something isolated, purely individual, and divorced from a relational dimension. We would not understand why Ivan Ilyich[10] looks at his wife and daughter with such hatred in his eyes. It cannot be that it is only because apparently for them it is as if he were already dead.

In actual fact such patients begin to feel that they have bodies, that is, that they only exist when they see themselves mirrored ("touched") in the other's desire. But it is also something they fear greatly. That is why it happens very quickly that the other's gaze becomes dehumanized, turning back into something mechanical. No longer an eager, vague gaze but the cold eye of a camera. The necrophilic urge that is so clearly captured in the works of Malani and McQueen in particular – but which is, after all, present in all the works of art we have examined so closely – reflects this constitutive dissent of the psyche, which turns into pathology when it cannot achieve balance.

The tropes of danger, trauma, mourning, and cruelty that the art of the sublime so effectively subjects us to, in short, make "palpable" to us how the many risks and distortions that go to make up the road to becoming human. The other essential point that the aesthetics of the sublime shows in such glaringly obvious fashion when seen this way is that this is not a road that one can travel alone. In other words, the clear and easy paradigm for understanding how the fabric of human subjectivity is woven can only be an intersubjective one and not a paradigm of the isolated subject. Equally modern is the accent on the pathetic element of the sublime, which anticipates the current theoretical emphasis on the role that emotions play in the processes of becoming subjects.

In short, it is a matter of developing a radically social theory of the emergence of the psyche. Yet also, and perhaps above all, it is a matter of extracting a coherent technique for treatment. Implicitly, we can also glean from it a theory of the essence of aesthetic experience *tout court*. In this sense any aesthetic experience has to do with the capacity that in *Beyond the Pleasure Principle* Freud[11] assigns to the dream – but which we now always see as composed of an intersubjective fabric – to transform fright (*Schreck*) into anguish (*Angst*). The negativity of the fright – which one is unprepared for and which risks causing a wound in the psychic skin –becomes a source of pleasure if one can distance oneself from it. It is essential to move away from pain. For this reason, regardless of scale, and as the aesthetics of the sublime reinterpreted in the light of the psychoanalytic concept of sublimation shows in exemplary fashion, pleasure is always a negative pleasure.

Notes

1 E. Dickinson, https://en.wikisource.org/wiki/That_odd_old_man_is_dead_a_year_(accessed Dec. 5th, 2022).
2 B.-C. Han, *Saving Beauty*, cited, p. 22.
3 F. Lyotard, "Newman: The Instant", cited, p. 245.
4 B. Newman, *The Sublime is Now*, cited.
5 F. Lyotard, "Newman: The Instant", cited, p. 246. According to T. Reik, *Der überraschte Psychologe. Über Erraten und Verstehen unbewusster Vorgänge*, A.W. Sijthoff's Uitgeversmaatschappij N J, Leiden 1935, the experience of surprise "emerges apparently directly and without preparation [*unmittelbar oder unvorbereitet*] and is accompanied by a special clarity [*besonderen Klarheit*]". Both qualities are explained by the decisive part that the unconscious plays in it.
6 T. Mann, *The Magic Mountain*, transl. by H. T. Lowe-Porter, A. Wheaton & Co., Exeter, 1924, p. 494, https://archive.org/details/in.ernet.dli.2015.2424/page/n503/mode/2up?q=bones+ (accessed Dec. 5th, 2022).
7 See A. Lemma, "Whose skin is it anyway? Some reflections on the psychic function of necrophilic fantasies", *Rivista di Psicoanalisi*, 59, 283–304, 2013.
8 See J. Kristeva, *Revolution in Poetic Language*, 1974, transl. by M. Waller, Columbia University Press, New York, 1984, about the perversion

inherent in language. According to the author, the sublimatory process already lies in the constitution of language as an "objet de type pervers" ("L'impudence d'énoncer: la langue maternelle", *Revue Française de Psychanalyse* 69, 1655–1667, 2005, p. 1658), i.e. removed from "normal" instinctual realization. By agreeing to abide by the rules of language, and thus by transfusing the drive into vocabulary and syntax, that is, by sexualising language, the subject frees himself from dependence on the real object. The basic idea, then, is that subjectivity is based on the constitutive cultural perversion that is the outcome of sublimation.

9 E. Sechaud, "Perdre, sublimer", *Revue Française de Psychanalyse*, 69, 1309–1379, 2005, p. 1345.

10 L. Tolstoy, *The Death of Ivan Ilyich*, 1886, transl. by L. Solotaroff, Bantam Classic, New York, 2004.

11 S. Freud, *Beyond the Pleasure Principle*, cited.

Index

Note: Page numbers in *italics* refer to figures and those followed by "n" refer to notes.